Understanding
Blood Pressure

Professor D.G. Beevers

Pub
in a

Family Doctor Publications, PO Box 4664, Poole, Dorset BH15 1NN

ISBN-13: 978 1 903474 30 3
ISBN-10: 1 903474 30 2

19992013

Contents

About the author

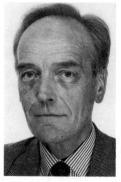

Professor D.G. Beevers, MD, FRCP is Emeritus Professor of Medicine, University of Birmingham. From 1977 to 2011 he was an Honorary Consultant Physician to the City Hospital, Birmingham. He is a founder committee member and past president of the British Hypertension Society and the Founding Editor of the *Journal of Human Hypertension*. His main interests are in clinical aspects of raised blood pressure and the importance of a population-based approach. In close collaboration with obstetricians, he has for many years run an antenatal hypertension clinic.

Introduction

How common is high blood pressure?

If you are over the age of 30 and can't remember when you last had your blood pressure checked then you ought to go and see your doctor. You could be one of the seven to ten million people in this country who have high blood pressure. Doctors usually use the term 'hypertension' to describe this condition which may cause no symptoms at all for very many years, but could eventually lead to serious complications, including heart disease and strokes.

In this book, the word hypertension is used to mean a blood pressure level that has been found on several separate occasions to be above normal, and that needs to be treated to prevent complications developing in the long term.

Who has high blood pressure?

The condition is very common (10 to 20 per cent of the population) in the UK and, the older you are, the more likely you are to have developed it. Whether you do so depends on a number of related factors, including:

- heredity – if your parents have high blood pressure there is a strong chance you have it too

- your diet – and especially the amounts of salt and alcohol that you consume

- your ethnic background

- whether you have diabetes

- whether you are overweight

- whether you take regular exercise.

How is high blood pressure diagnosed?

If all this sounds alarming, there is good news too. Hypertension can be easily diagnosed: your blood pressure can be measured quickly and painlessly at your GP's surgery or health centre. When the reading is above normal, the check can be repeated three or four times if necessary to establish that the first figure wasn't a chance finding.

How is high blood pressure treated?

Even if you do have hypertension, you may be one of the many people who don't need drug treatment for some time (and possibly not ever), provided that you make some straightforward lifestyle changes that will not only lower your blood pressure but bring general health benefits too.

When treatment is required, there are a number of very effective drugs available, which are taken in tablet form, usually once daily. Most people find that they have no problems at all with the treatment, but, if you do experience side effects from one drug, there are usually other, equally effective alternatives.

More modern drugs tend to have very few side effects. Research has shown that controlling hypertension with drug therapy can bring down the risk of a stroke by 35 to 40 per cent, and the risk of coronary heart disease by 20 to 25 per cent.

A symptomless disease

The most important message on hypertension is that you may not know that you have it until it has done you serious damage, unless you have your blood pressure checked. Even quite seriously raised blood pressure can be controlled once it is identified and, provided that you keep taking the treatment prescribed for you and have regular check-ups, your chances of developing serious and potentially life-threatening complications are dramatically reduced.

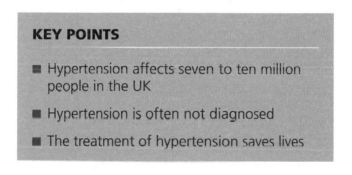

KEY POINTS

- Hypertension affects seven to ten million people in the UK

- Hypertension is often not diagnosed

- The treatment of hypertension saves lives

What is blood pressure?

Blood pressure

When doctors talk about blood pressure, what they mean is the pressure within the large blood vessels as your heart forces blood to circulate around your body. On the whole, the lower your blood pressure, the healthier you are in the long term (except in some very rare conditions in which excessively low blood pressure is part of an underlying disease).

Blood pressure

Blood pressure is the pressure within the arteries as the heart forces blood to circulate around your body.

Elastic artery wall

Blood pressure wave from beat of heart

Greater pressure

Lower pressure

The circulatory system

Blood picks up oxygen in the lungs from the air that we breathe in. This oxygenated blood enters the heart and is then pumped out to all parts of the body in blood vessels called arteries. Larger blood vessels branch into smaller and smaller ones and then to microscopic arterioles, which eventually link to tiny networks of blood vessels known as capillaries.

This network of larger arteries, medium-sized arterioles and tiny capillaries allows blood to reach every cell of the body and deposit its oxygen, which is used by the cells to make the vital energy that they need to survive.

Once the blood has deposited its oxygen in the cells, the deoxygenated blood returns to the heart in the veins, to be pumped back up to the lungs to pick up more oxygen.

During each heartbeat, the heart muscle contracts to push blood around the body. The pressure produced by the heart is highest when it contracts, and this is known as the systolic (higher value) pressure. Then the heart muscle relaxes before its next contraction, and the pressure is at its lowest, which is known as the diastolic (lower value) pressure. Both systolic and diastolic pressures are measured when you have your blood pressure checked.

The dividing line between a normal and an abnormal blood pressure is not easy to define. Perhaps the best definition is that level of blood pressure above which treatment has been shown to be worthwhile (see page 27).

Cardiovascular system

Diagram showing the heart and circulation with veins (blue) draining the blood back to the heart where it is pumped to the lungs and back to the rest of the body through the arteries (red). Larger blood vessels branch into smaller and smaller ones and then to tiny networks of blood vessels known as capillaries, where oxygen and nutrients are passed from the blood into the surrounding cells.

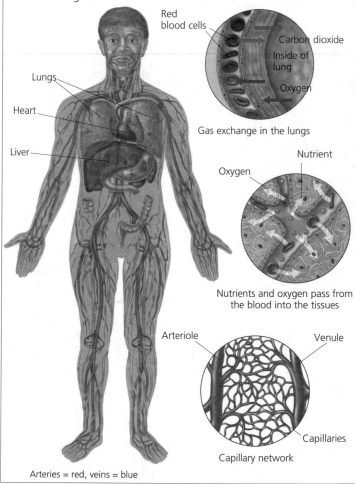

Red blood cells

Carbon dioxide

Inside of lung

Oxygen

Gas exchange in the lungs

Lungs

Heart

Liver

Nutrient

Oxygen

Nutrients and oxygen pass from the blood into the tissues

Arteriole

Venule

Capillaries

Capillary network

Arteries = red, veins = blue

The sequence that makes up a heartbeat

The heartbeat sequence has three phases. The timing of these phases must be accurately maintained regardless of how slowly or rapidly the heart is beating.

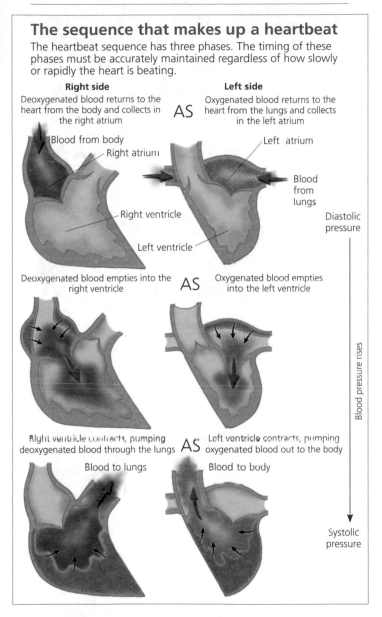

Right side

Deoxygenated blood returns to the heart from the body and collects in the right atrium

Left side

Oxygenated blood returns to the heart from the lungs and collects in the left atrium

AS

Blood from body

Right atrium

Left atrium

Blood from lungs

Right ventricle

Left ventricle

Diastolic pressure

Deoxygenated blood empties into the right ventricle

AS

Oxygenated blood empties into the left ventricle

Blood pressure rises

Right ventricle contracts, pumping deoxygenated blood through the lungs

AS

Left ventricle contracts, pumping oxygenated blood out to the body

Blood to lungs

Blood to body

Systolic pressure

What determines blood pressure?

The blood pressure is determined by:

- The pumping strength of each heartbeat – the greater the strength the higher the blood pressure
- The volume of blood in the circulation – a greater volume of blood will increase blood pressure
- The diameter of the blood vessels – narrower blood vessels raise blood pressure

KEY POINTS

- High blood pressure is caused by a narrowing of the microscopic arterioles in all tissues

- Systolic pressure is the pressure in the larger vessels when the heart contracts

- Diastolic pressure is the pressure when the heart relaxes between beats

Measuring your blood pressure

How often should blood pressure be measured?

Most people have had their blood pressure taken at least once – perhaps by the doctor or nurse at the surgery, in hospital or, in the case of a pregnant woman, at the antenatal clinic. You may possibly have opted to have it done at a pharmacy or health food shop or even have tried taking it yourself using one of the special kits that can be bought over the counter.

Around 30 per cent of the adult population have, however, never had their blood pressure measured, usually because they feel entirely well and have not needed to visit their doctors. As raised blood pressure is usually a symptomless condition, many of these people will be found to have raised blood pressure if they undergo a routine check. It is now recommended that all adults should have their blood pressure checked at least once every five years. If the blood pressure is not entirely normal, more frequent checks are necessary.

How is blood pressure measured?

Although the ideal method would be to measure the blood pressure actually inside the arteries, this is clearly not feasible on a large scale because it would involve needles. However, an accurate reflection of the pressure under which blood is being pumped can be obtained using a less invasive approach. Usually you will be asked to sit down and the person performing the check wraps a rubber-lined cuff, which is part of the pressure-measuring device known as a sphygmomanometer, around your upper arm.

Determining systolic blood pressure

The cuff is inflated, either with a small hand pump or automatically by an electronic measuring device. This will stop the blood flow to your arm temporarily. The cuff is then deflated slowly until the pressure is low enough for blood to start to pass under the cuff. Electronic blood pressure measurement devices can detect this blood flow. Very occasionally, the doctor or nurse may listen with a stethoscope over the artery just below the cuff and hear the sounds as blood starts to flow.

Determining diastolic blood pressure

As the cuff continues to deflate turbulence occurs in the underlying artery because it is only partially blocked. Finally, the cuff will reach the pressure where there is no narrowing of the underlying artery and at this stage the electronic manometers (pressure-measuring device) can detect the absence of any turbulence. Alternatively, a doctor or nurse will note that turbulence sounds have disappeared.

The pressure where blood first starts to pass under the cuff is called the systolic blood pressure and the pressure where there is no turbulence in the artery, because the cuff pressure is low, is called the diastolic blood pressure. The systolic blood pressure coincides with the maximum pressure within the arterial tree and the diastolic blood pressure coincides with the minimum blood pressure in the system.

Measurement problems

This technique of measuring blood pressure is indirect but has the benefit of being easy to perform. There are, however, four sources of error when blood pressure is measured in this way.

The patient

Falsely raised blood pressures will occur if the patient is very anxious or involved in any animated conversation. This sort of error can be minimised if blood pressure is taken in a very quiet and peaceful environment. Sometimes the first reading of blood pressure may be raised, but the second or third readings may settle considerably as the patient becomes familiar with the technique.

Any interaction between the patient and the observer can raise the blood pressure in the short term. In particular, a substantial rise in blood pressure can occur when it is measured either by a doctor or, to a lesser extent, by a nurse. This is sometimes called the 'white coat effect'.

The observer

Observer error was mainly a problem with the old-fashioned method of measuring blood pressure using a stethoscope and mercury column. This is because the decision about whether the doctor or nurse can

How is blood pressure measured?

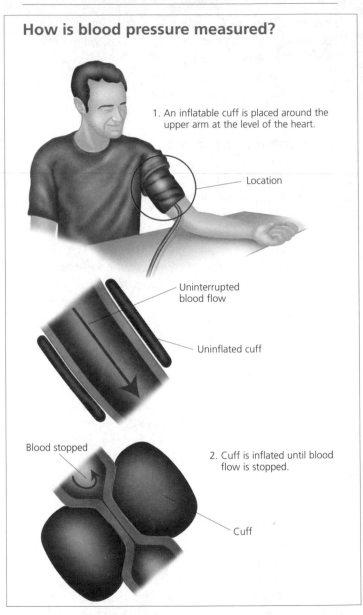

1. An inflatable cuff is placed around the upper arm at the level of the heart.

Location

Uninterrupted blood flow

Uninflated cuff

Blood stopped

2. Cuff is inflated until blood flow is stopped.

Cuff

How is blood pressure measured? (contd)

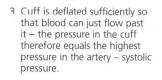

3. Cuff is deflated sufficiently so that blood can just flow past it – the pressure in the cuff therefore equals the highest pressure in the artery – systolic pressure.

4. As cuff is further deflated turbulent blood flow occurs in the artery, which can be detected.

Turbulence

5. Cuff is deflated until there are no turbulence sounds – now the pressure in the cuff equals the lowest pressure in the artery – diastolic pressure.

Uninterrupted blood flow

hear the systolic and diastolic sounds is subjective and open to error or bias. Unfortunately the quality of measurement by some doctors and nurses is extremely poor, leading to serious overestimation of the blood pressure.

The cuff

If the cuff is too small the blood pressure is overestimated. It is also very important that the cuff be at exactly the same level as the heart. If the cuff is above the level of the heart, the blood pressure will be underestimated, and if below the blood pressure will be overestimated.

The manometer

Both the electronic and the mercury blood pressure-measuring systems must be accurate. Most electronic machines marketed nowadays have passed criteria laid down by the British Hypertension Society (BHS). It is important that only manometers that have been passed by the BHS are used. Mercury machines can deteriorate if they are not maintained regularly.

In a small number of patients it proves impossible to measure blood pressure using electronic blood pressure-measuring devices. Under these circumstances the doctor or nurse will have to use a mercury manometer. Measurement of blood pressure using a reliable mercury system remains the 'gold standard', but the advent of automatic and semi-automatic systems means that mercury manometers are now rarely needed. All general practitioner health centres and hospital outpatient clinics will need to have one well-maintained mercury manometer available whereas there should be semi-automatic machines in every clinical room.

Measuring blood pressure

The mercury manometer is the traditional method for measuring blood pressure. Electronic measuring devices mean that mercury manometers are now rarely needed.

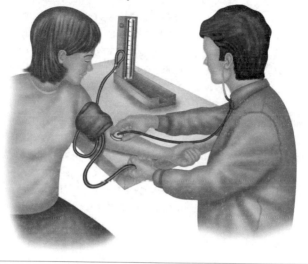

An important advantage of the electronic blood pressure equipment is that the clinician can effortlessly take several readings and obtain a truer picture of the real blood pressure as the patient becomes familiar with the technique. It is increasingly felt that a hurried one-off blood pressure reading measured with a mercury manometer is of little clinical value. Blood pressures that are raised should be re-checked and many settle over five to ten minutes.

Taking a blood pressure reading

Usually, you will be asked to sit down and the cuff is applied to your upper arm so that it is at the same level as your heart. It is very important that you are as relaxed as possible and that your arm is supported by resting your elbow on a table – the effort of holding it up could otherwise produce a falsely high reading.

Everyone's blood pressure is immensely variable and yours may go up if you're feeling anxious or stressed, so try to relax as much as you can while it's being measured. Your doctor or nurse will probably take the first reading as a rough guide and take a second measurement to get the actual reading. If your blood pressure is clearly settling to a lower level between the first and second reading, you may need to have a third or even a fourth reading at another visit to the clinic some days or weeks later to make sure that the final figure is a truly representative value. This is particularly important if the finding on the first or second measurement is only slightly above normal. There is evidence to suggest that, in most people, the blood pressure 'bottoms out' at the fourth visit, with little further fall after that. There are, however, many exceptions to this rule.

Which arm should be used?

Blood pressure should be checked initially in both arms, and thereafter, if there is no important difference between the arms, the nearest arm can be used. Important differences between the arms are found in about 10 per cent of the population. If there is a difference, then the blood pressure should be measured in the arm with the highest pressure. This is more common in older patients and may be the result of narrowing of blood vessels in the arm (see page 28).

If your upper arm is larger than average (more than 33 centimetres around), the person measuring your blood pressure will need to use a larger cuff, otherwise there may be a falsely high reading. About 15 per cent of people with high blood pressure have an arm circumference that is greater than 33 centimetres, so it is crucially important that the correct size of cuff is used.

Standing up, sitting down or lying?

It is not usual to be asked to stand up to have your blood pressure checked because it's more difficult to provide support for your arm. There are some occasions when it is done – for example, in people with diabetes, and in elderly people or anyone who experiences dizziness or other symptoms on standing. The former is because the blood pressure of people with diabetes may fall when they stand. Normally, there is no significant change in blood pressure on standing up but in certain conditions, including diabetes, this can occur, and is referred to as postural hypotension. It may or may not be associated with dizziness. There is no point in measuring blood pressure lying down; all the clinical research into hypertension and its treatment has relied on seated pressure recordings.

Systolic and diastolic blood pressure

As we have seen, measuring blood pressure involves recording both the highest (systolic) and the lowest (diastolic) levels in your system, so the reading will record two figures. Conventionally, blood pressure is expressed as systolic pressure over diastolic pressure, for example, 140/94 mmHg (millimetres of mercury).

140

Systolic pressure
The pressure produced in the circulation when the heart contracts

94

Diastolic pressure
The pressure in the circulation between heartbeats

The relative importance of systolic and diastolic blood pressure has been the subject of much research. In fact, contrary to what most people believe, over the age of 40 the systolic pressure is more important than the diastolic when it comes to predicting who will and who will not develop heart disease. The problem is that everyone's systolic blood pressure varies considerably, and this is even more so with older people.

The importance of systolic blood pressure has recently been emphasised by the publication of two reliable studies which showed that reducing the systolic pressure was worthwhile in people whose diastolic blood pressure was normal or even below normal. This condition is known medically as isolated systolic hypertension (ISH). It mostly affects people over the age of 65 and, if it is not treated, they are at high risk of developing heart disease or stroke.

In general, the lower your blood pressure readings, the better. When treating high blood pressure, the aim is to reduce all risk factors for heart disease such as smoking, blood cholesterol levels, and to keep blood pressure under 140/80 mmHg.

'White coat' hypertension

'White coat' and 'office' hypertension are terms applied to those people whose blood pressure is raised only when they are seeing a doctor. In recent years, it has become possible to record blood pressure over 24-hour periods at home (using automatic electronic equipment), and this has shown that many people's blood pressure goes back down to the normal range within an hour or so of leaving the surgery or hospital. When this happens, the person is said to have 'white coat' hypertension. The technique for detecting white coat hypertension is called 24-hour ambulatory blood pressure monitoring (ABPM).

The exact significance of white coat hypertension has, until recently, been the source of much debate. Now, however there are several long-term follow-up studies of thousands of people who have had their blood pressure measured both in a clinical setting and by 24-hour ambulatory monitoring. It has become clear that people whose pressures are raised in the clinic but absolutely normal for the remaining 23 hours of the day have the same risk of stroke or heart attack as those whose pressures are quite normal all the time. 'White coat' hypertension, at least in the short term, is not a serious condition. On a much longer, five to ten years, basis some people with 'white coat' hypertension may develop persistent hypertension both in the clinic and at home. So if you are diagnosed as having 'white coat' hypertension and deemed not to need blood pressure-lowering drugs, you should be reviewed by your doctor or clinic nurse about once a year.

The findings described above prompted the National Institute for Health and Clinical Excellence (NICE) and the British Hypertension Society (BHS) to publish new guidelines in August 2011). They now recommend that all people whose blood pressures are mildly of moderately raised should undergo ABPM in order to see whether their blood pressure settles to normal once they are away from the GP health centre or the clinic. They regard the 24-hour ambulatory blood pressure as the gold standard for assessing the need for treatment.

24-hour ambulatory blood pressure monitoring (ABPM)

Some of the larger GP health centres have their own equipment to do ABPM. Some of the smaller practices may opt to refer to the cardiology outpatient department at your local hospital. Wherever the ABPM is done, you will need to attend on two consecutive mornings, each appointment lasting for about half an hour.

On the first morning the technician or nurse will attach a cuff to your left upper arm if you are right handed or your right arm if you are left handed. The rubber tube from the cuff is then fitted under your shirt or top and attached to a monitor, which is about the size of a paperback book (although a little heavier) attached to your belt. The monitor is switched on to take the first recording in the clinic. You will then be able to leave the clinic and go about your normal everyday business. The cuff will inflate automatically every half-hour. When you feel the cuff inflating, try to keep your arm as still as possible. You will, however, be able to do all daily tasks including driving. The only thing you can't do is have a bath or shower.

Contrary to what one might expect, this blood pressure monitoring is very well tolerated by the vast majority of people. Very few people find that it interferes with their daily activities. Similarly very few people find that it affects their sleeping. However, if you feel that the cuff inflation does interfere with sleeping, you must tell the clinic staff when you return the next morning. Overnight blood pressures are very important. If your blood pressure does not settle when you are asleep you may be classified as a 'non-dipper'. Non-dippers are known to have a greater chance of

Ambulatory blood pressure monitoring

Ambulatory blood pressure monitoring (ABPM) is when your blood pressure is being measured as you move around, living your normal daily life.

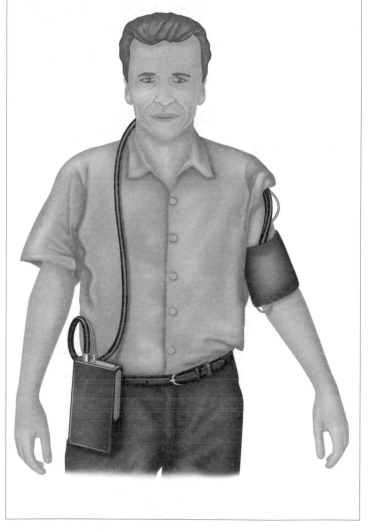

developing a heart attack or stroke. However, if you had a disturbed night, the failure of the blood pressure to settle may be less important.

Twenty-four hours after the monitor was fitted you should return to the clinic to have it removed. The clinic staff will then decode the monitor to produce a computerised report. This will include every individual pressure reading, as well as the daytime and night-time average pressures. Some clinic staff will give you a copy of the report but others may prefer to send the report to your doctor so that you can discuss it in more detail.

Home blood pressure measurement (HBPM)

A reasonable alternative to 24-hour ABPM is home self-monitoring of blood pressure. However, there is as yet less information on the long-term significance of measuring blood pressures in this way; 24-hour ABPM remains the gold standard, but it is the practice of this author to recommend that all people with raised blood pressure should monitor their own pressure at home.

Home blood pressure monitors cost around £20. Most are reliable and accurate. It is best to purchase monitors that are endorsed by the BHS. If in doubt it would be worthwhile to take your monitor with you when you next see your doctor. It will then be possible to check your monitor against the clinic readings.

You should not purchase home monitors that are supplied with wrist cuffs or even finger cuffs. The accuracy of this method of measuring blood pressure is questionable, because it is important that the cuff is at the same level as your heart which is difficult to standardise with wrist monitors.

Home monitoring should be carried out in a quiet room, preferably with no one else there. Do not measure blood pressure if you are under stress or in any discomfort. Apply the cuff to your upper arm just as in the clinic. If you have an arm circumference of more than 33 centimetres you will need to buy a larger cuff. Make sure that your arm is resting on a table so that the cuff is level with your heart. Above all, be relaxed.

Automatic blood pressure machines

Electronic automatic blood pressure machines can be easy to use, but choose carefully to ensure accuracy.

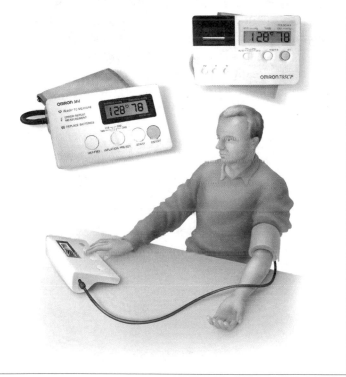

Switch on the monitor and after a few seconds press the start button. The cuff will inflate steadily and then deflate, and during deflation your blood pressure will be measured. Take a minimum of three recordings about 60 seconds apart. If the pressure was raised at the first reading but continues to settle with repeated measures, it may be useful to take a fourth or even fifth reading.

Measure your blood pressure sometimes in the morning, sometimes in the afternoon and sometimes in the evening. You will then obtain a 'picture' of your pressure throughout the day.

Above all it is important to write down all blood pressure readings together with the date and time. It is best to buy a small exercise book to keep all the measurements. When you consult your doctor or practice nurse, take your exercise book with you. Your home readings are more important than those measured in the clinic.

KEY POINTS

- It is important that you are totally relaxed when your blood pressure is being measured

- Systolic blood pressure is now known to be as important as, or even more important than, diastolic pressure

- Automatic measuring systems can be employed to measure blood pressure away from the clinic or health centre

What is hypertension and why does it matter?

Diagnosing hypertension

There are two thresholds for classifying you as having hypertension of a level that requires blood pressure-lowering drugs. These take into account your total cardiovascular risk of developing a heart attack or a stroke. In high-risk individuals with existing damage to their blood vessels or with diabetes, the threshold is 140/90 mmHg. In all other people who are at low risk, with no other medical problems, the threshold is 160/100 mmHg. These thresholds may change as more research becomes available.

There is a strong tendency for blood pressure to rise with advancing age. Thus, hypertension of a level where treatment would be considered necessary occurs in 10 to 20 per cent of patients aged 20 years. However, up to 60 per cent of patients over the age of 60 require treatment. For this reason blood pressures that are below 140/90 mmHg but above 120/80 mmHg are sometimes classified as being 'high–normal' or 'pre-hypertensive'. This is because a very large proportion of such people will develop mild hypertension in the subsequent years.

Defining hypertension

Blood pressure readings are a remarkably accurate predictor of life expectancy: the higher the pressure the greater the risk. Even people whose blood pressures are average for the population have a slightly greater risk of heart disease than people with lower than average. For this reason it has been extremely difficult to find a simple working definition of hypertension. Perhaps the most sensible view is to define it as:

> 'That level of blood pressure where treatment with antihypertensive drugs does more good than harm.'

If your blood pressure is more than 160/100 mmHg, and if you have several different risk factors for heart disease, such as high cholesterol, being a smoker and a family tendency to heart disease, then treating your high blood pressure is very worthwhile. (This is explained in detail in the section beginning on page 85.)

On the other hand, for some young people with only very marginally raised blood pressure, and no other risk factors for heart disease, the value of blood pressure-lowering drugs is very small and drug treatment may be held back. It is, however, crucial that such people are re-checked at intervals of roughly six months.

The silent killer

Hypertension has been called the 'silent killer' because it usually causes no symptoms until a late stage of the disease. Contrary to what many people believe, it is not possible to feel your own blood pressure. The only way to find out whether your blood pressure is raised or not is to have it measured with a blood pressure machine – see pages 9–24.

As hypertension causes no symptoms until complications begin to show themselves, about half of all those who have it are unaware that they do. The only solution for this problem is for all adults to attend their family doctor for a routine check.

Why does hypertension matter?

Blood vessels are like rubber tubes that carry blood constantly to wherever it is needed. Arteries, which carry blood out of the heart, have to withstand the great pressures with which the blood is pumped out of the heart. If the blood pressure is higher than usual over many years, as in untreated hypertension, the vessels get damaged. The lining of the arteries can become roughened and thickened, and this eventually causes them to narrow and become less flexible, or elastic, than previously. In addition, the arteries become silted up with a fatty substance called atheroma.

If an artery gets too narrow, blood can't get through properly, and the part of the body that relies on that artery for its blood supply is starved of blood and the all-important oxygen that it carries. As the artery narrows there is an increased tendency to develop blood clots (thrombosis) over the area of atheroma, which may cause total blockage of the artery, so that the part of the body that it serves dies. The dead area of the heart or brain is called an infarct.

Other risk factors

High blood pressure over many years can cause all these problems and the whole point of measuring blood pressure regularly, and treating it effectively if it is high, is to prevent these complications. However, you are more likely to develop these complications if you smoke and if you have untreated high blood cholesterol levels. The reason is that cigarette smoking damages blood vessels in much the same way that high blood pressure does, making the artery itself stiffer and narrower, and its lining thick and rough.

High cholesterol also causes deposits of atheroma in the lining of the artery. When this 'furring up' process occurs in the arteries that supply the heart muscle it is called coronary heart disease (CHD). This furring up process also occurs in the blood vessels supplying the brain. As with blood pressure it is not possible for your level of serum cholesterol to be too low, and similarly treatment to lower cholesterol also saves lives.

Another common risk factor that can also contribute to narrowing of the arteries in the heart, brain and lower limbs is diabetes (type 2 diabetes mellitus) which affects 4 to 5 per cent of the white population and 10 to 15 per cent of the south Asian and African–Caribbean populations in the UK. High glucose levels in the blood damage arteries in a similar way to high blood pressure.

Type 1 diabetes mellitus usually occurs in younger people, who are more prone to develop kidney disease and damage to their retinas. Almost all those with type 1 diabetes have raised blood pressure.

Coronary thrombosis

A coronary thrombosis occurs when a clot forms in the coronary arteries that supply blood to the heart muscle. In a heart attack a clot typically forms on a break in the fibrous plaque in a diseased vessel.

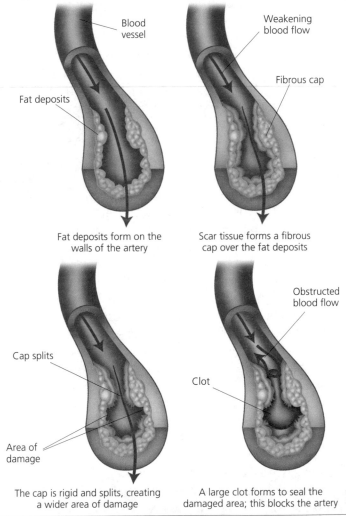

Blood vessel

Fat deposits

Fat deposits form on the walls of the artery

Weakening blood flow

Fibrous cap

Scar tissue forms a fibrous cap over the fat deposits

Cap splits

Area of damage

The cap is rigid and splits, creating a wider area of damage

Obstructed blood flow

Clot

A large clot forms to seal the damaged area; this blocks the artery

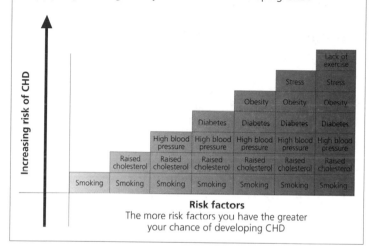

Risk factors for coronary heart disease (CHD)

Several factors have been found to influence an individual's risk of developing CHD. The greater the number of risk factors that apply to you, the greater your chance of developing CHD.

Increasing risk of CHD

						Lack of exercise
					Stress	Stress
				Obesity	Obesity	Obesity
			Diabetes	Diabetes	Diabetes	Diabetes
		High blood pressure	High blood pressure	High blood pressure	High blood pressure	High blood pressure
	Raised cholesterol	Raised cholesterol	Raised cholesterol	Raised cholesterol	Raised cholesterol	Raised cholesterol
Smoking	Smoking	Smoking	Smoking	Smoking	Smoking	Smoking

Risk factors
The more risk factors you have the greater your chance of developing CHD

There is now increasing awareness that people whose kidneys are not functioning as well as they should have a marked increase in their risk of developing a heart attack or a stroke over the coming years. These newly recognised high-risk patients need careful attention with accurate control of both blood pressure and blood cholesterol levels.

It wouldn't do to paint too gloomy a picture, however. The whole point of checking blood pressure is that, if you are found to have hypertension, it is possible to treat it effectively and so bring your risk of heart disease and strokes back down to normal. It doesn't matter particularly how severe the hypertension was in the first place. What really matters is how well your blood pressure is controlled over the ensuing years.

It's better to have had severe hypertension that has been well treated than to have slightly raised blood pressure that remains untreated or neglected.

Long-term effects of high blood pressure

Although there are many possible, serious, long-term effects of high blood pressure, it must be stressed that all these complications can be prevented with effective antihypertensive treatment.

Angina

The heart is a muscle like any other that needs its own blood supply, which is brought to it by the coronary arteries. If these coronary arteries narrow, blood doesn't get to the heart muscle efficiently. So when the heart needs to work a bit harder than usual, like when you are walking up a hill, the heart muscle cannot get the blood supply and oxygen that it needs. This causes pain in the chest, known as myocardial ischaemia or angina.

Heart attack

If a coronary artery narrows and then a blood clot forms, leading to total blockage, the part of the heart muscle that relies on that coronary artery dies. This is known as a coronary thrombosis, leading to a myocardial infarction or a heart attack. The most common symptom of this is crushing pain across the front of the chest.

Heart failure and breathlessness

Over the years, as arteries narrow and become less elastic as a result of hypertension, it gets harder and

Changes causing angina or heart attack

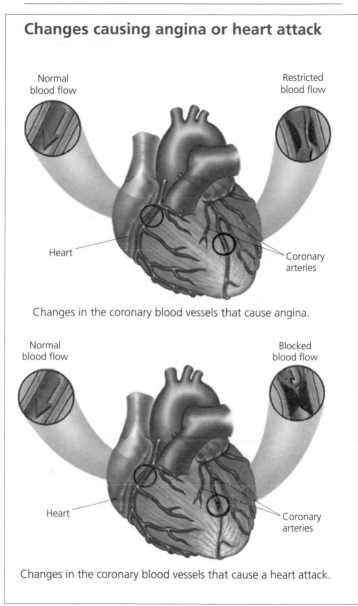

Normal blood flow

Restricted blood flow

Heart

Coronary arteries

Changes in the coronary blood vessels that cause angina.

Normal blood flow

Blocked blood flow

Heart

Coronary arteries

Changes in the coronary blood vessels that cause a heart attack.

Heart failure and breathlessness

Excessive fluid flows out of the blood into lung tissue, where it collects causing breathlessness.

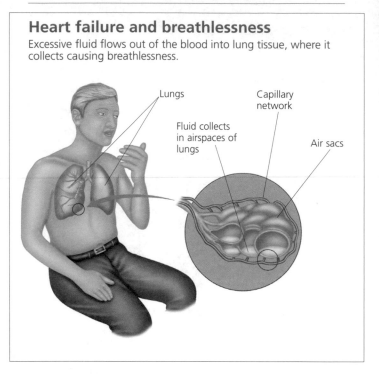

Lungs

Capillary network

Fluid collects in airspaces of lungs

Air sacs

harder for the heart to pump blood out efficiently to the rest of the body. The increased workload eventually damages the heart and impairs its performance. Fluid collects in the lungs, causing shortness of breath, particularly when lying flat. This is known as left heart failure or left ventricular failure (LVF).

Irregular heart beats

High blood pressure increases the chances of developing a fast irregular heart rhythm called atrial fibrillation. This risk is even greater if the alcohol intake is more than 10 drinks per week. Atrial fibrillation itself is an important cause of strokes.

Stroke

Narrowing of an artery that carries blood and oxygen to the brain can lead to temporary loss of function in the part of the brain served by that artery; this is known as a transient ischaemic attack (TIA). Permanent closing off of the artery with a blood clot results in the death of the part of the brain reliant on that artery, which results in a cerebral infarction causing a stroke. Less commonly, the blood vessels in the brain may rupture, leading to a brain haemorrhage (intracerebral haemorrhage).

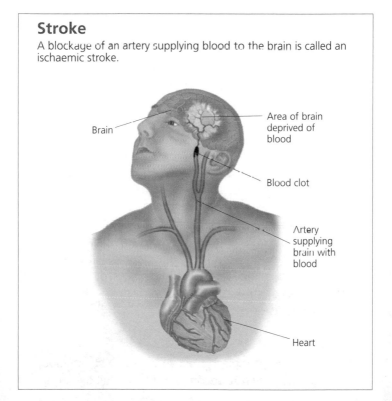

Stroke

A blockage of an artery supplying blood to the brain is called an ischaemic stroke.

Brain

Area of brain deprived of blood

Blood clot

Artery supplying brain with blood

Heart

Dementia

People with neglected, longstanding hypertension are at increased risk of developing dementia or cognitive decline, with reduced short-term memory and increasing forgetfulness. No dedicated long-term treatment study has been carried out to test whether lowering blood pressure reduces dementia, although one reliable trial in elderly patients did show some evidence of dementia prevention.

Peripheral artery disease

The major blood vessels in the legs can be damaged, resulting in less blood flow and cause pain in the calf muscles on walking. This is called intermittent claudication. In addition, narrowing or blockage of the very small arteries in the feet can cause loss of the toes due to gangrene. This is particularly a problem in people with diabetes.

Kidney damage

When blood vessels supplying the kidneys are affected the result may be gradual kidney damage, which affects how the body gets rid of waste products, including drugs. This is why a blood test to check kidney function (serum creatinine levels) is a vital part of regular check-ups for anyone with hypertension. As stated earlier, there is increasing information that people with even mild kidney damage have a greatly increased risk of heart attacks or strokes. The reasons for this are not as yet fully understood.

Eye damage

The small blood vessels in the eyes can also be affected, although this may not become apparent until damage

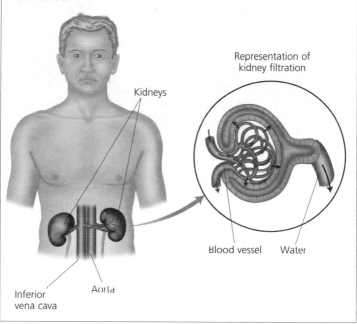

Kidney damage

There are usually two kidneys; their function is to excrete urine and to regulate the water, electrolyte composition and acidity of the blood.

Representation of kidney filtration

Kidneys

Blood vessel   Water

Inferior vena cava

Aorta

is extensive. Very rarely, in very severe hypertension, there may be damage to the retina with haemorrhages, infarcts and swelling of the optic nerve. This condition is still called malignant hypertension, although nowadays with treatment the outlook is very good.

KEY POINTS

■ High blood pressure is one of the three risk factors for heart attack and stroke

■ The other factors are smoking and raised blood cholesterol levels

■ Lowering blood pressure (and lowering blood cholesterol) saves lives

What causes hypertension?

Categorising hypertension

In 95 per cent of cases there is no specific underlying cause, and this condition is known as primary or essential hypertension. The remaining five per cent of people have a problem with their kidneys or adrenal glands, located at the top of the kidneys, which causes their hypertension. Doctors refer to this as secondary hypertension.

Risk factors for high blood pressure

There are a number of different factors that may contribute to causing raised blood pressure. Heredity plays a part which means that hypertension can run in families. Blood pressure tends to increase with age but this is partly because of changes in lifestyle; many people put on weight and get less active as they get older and both these factors may contribute to the development of hypertension. More importantly, the rise in pressure with age is greater in people who eat a lot of salty foods.

Risk factors for cardiovascular damage

Modifiable (we can change)	Non-modifiable (we cannot change)
• Smoking • Raised cholesterol • Diabetes • Obesity • Stress • Lack of exercise • Diet – salt • Alcohol	• Genetic factors, e.g. an inherited high cholesterol level • Gender – more men than women get high blood pressure • Age • Racial background

Racial background plays a part, with people of African–Caribbean origin living in western societies having a higher prevalence of hypertension than white people. This is probably because African–Caribbean people handle salt in the body differently from other groups. However, migration studies show that, although racial origins do play a part, it is the diet and other lifestyle factors that are more significant. Anyone who lives in the more affluent western countries is more prone to hypertension than those who live in the rural areas of developing countries. This is probably because the western diet is high in calories, dairy products and salt, which with reduced exercise is causing the increasing epidemic of obesity, hypertension and diabetes. However as the people in developing countries change to a western style of foods and activity, their pressures rise. Hypertension is now very common in the towns and cities of Africa and Asia.

Blood pressure always varies throughout the day and is usually higher during exercise as the heart needs to pump blood around the body faster, although people who exercise regularly will tend to have lower blood pressures than non-active people when at rest. Your blood pressure is lower when you are sleeping or resting.

How does the body regulate blood pressure?
Sympathetic nervous system

There are two systems in the body that are involved in helping us to maintain normal blood pressures in all circumstances if possible. One is the sympathetic nervous system which releases chemicals such as adrenaline and noradrenaline; these can both open or vasodilate the microscopic arterioles and narrow them by vasoconstriction, as required, depending on which parts of our body need to be ready for action.

This system comes into operation to enable us to respond in a crisis by concentrating our physical resources where they are needed to help us survive a perceived threat. This means shutting down non-essential functions – such as digestion – for the duration of the crisis to prepare us to fight or run away. For early humans, this was essential when life was full of physical danger, but for most people today the system is likely to be triggered by emotional or psychological stress rather than by actual life-threatening situations most of the time. As a result of its narrowing effect on small blood vessels, this process can play a part in causing hypertension. Drugs that act on this system, for example, the alpha blockers and beta blockers, can therefore be used to control it.

Renin–angiotensin system

The other important system is an enzyme produced by the kidneys, known as renin, which activates a hormone called angiotensin II. Angiotensin II makes blood vessels constrict. Drugs that block angiotensin, called the angiotensin-converting enzyme (ACE) inhibitors and angiotensin receptor blockers (ARBs), can help to lower blood pressure.

Angiotensin also stimulates the release of a hormone called aldosterone from the adrenal glands. This hormone causes salt and water retention by the kidneys which may further elevate the blood pressure.

Calcium

The microscopic blood vessels, called arterioles, have smooth muscle cells in their walls which contract when calcium concentrations rise. People with hypertension have higher calcium levels in their smooth muscle cells than those with normal blood pressure, although it is still not known why. Calcium enters the cells through calcium channels.

In people with hypertension, it is thought that these rises in the calcium concentration cause the arterioles to constrict which makes it harder for the heart to pump blood through them. Long-term constriction of the arterioles is also thought to damage their walls, leading to further rises in blood pressure. Drugs that block the calcium channels (calcium channel blockers or CCBs, such as nifedipine) allow the arterioles to open up again which lowers blood pressure.

Although all the hormones mentioned here (renin, angiotensin, aldosterone, adrenaline and noradrenaline) play a role in regulating blood pressure in all people, it seems that people with high blood pressure are more

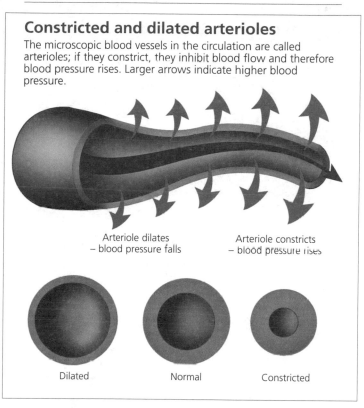

Constricted and dilated arterioles

The microscopic blood vessels in the circulation are called arterioles; if they constrict, they inhibit blood flow and therefore blood pressure rises. Larger arrows indicate higher blood pressure.

Arteriole dilates
– blood pressure falls

Arteriole constricts
– blood pressure rises

Dilated

Normal

Constricted

susceptible to their effects. People with hypertension do not have more of these hormones in their bloodstream, but blocking their effects with drugs lowers blood pressure only if it was raised in the first place.

The common pathway of all of these mechanisms is narrowing of the arterioles, causing increased resistance to blood flow. The heart continues to pump normally, so the pressure within the whole arterial system must rise.

Hypertension: problems throughout the circulation

Healthy artery walls are elastic, allowing the wall to flex with the blood pressure wave. If the wall stiffens, the ability to flex is lost and the pressure in the circulation will rise.

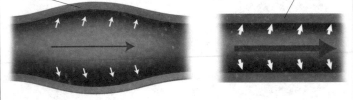

Flexible wall

Stiff wall

If the arterioles narrow, there is increased resistance to blood flow. The heart continues to pump normally, so the pressure within the circulation rises.

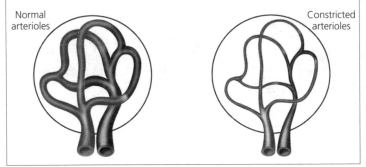

Normal arterioles

Constricted arterioles

Why your lifestyle matters

As far as you as an individual are concerned, your blood pressure level depends on the interplay of genetic or inherited factors and the influences of your lifestyle. Hypertension clearly runs in families and this holds true even after allowances have been made for the fact that families tend to share the same lifestyle and diet. Excellent research conducted among twins who were brought up separately or together, and also

The effect of sustained high blood pressure on the heart

With prolonged high blood pressure, the heart muscle gets thicker and more bulky as it works harder against the increased pressure. This thickened muscle is stiffer and functions less well than normal heart muscle.

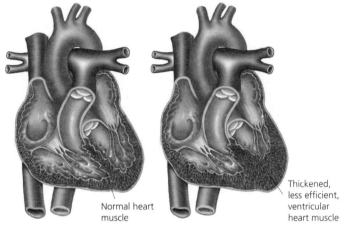

Normal heart muscle

Thickened, less efficient, ventricular heart muscle

among adopted children compared with non-adopted children, has been able to identify how much of the similarity in blood pressure within families is the result of inheritance compared with the proportion resulting from similarities in lifestyle. Roughly speaking, about half of all the variation in blood pressure between people is the result of genetic factors and half is the result of dietary factors dating back to early childhood.

Salt intake

Salt intake has a direct effect on blood pressure. It has been shown that the rise in blood pressure as we get older, which occurs in all urban societies, is partly the result of the amount of salt that we eat. Reducing

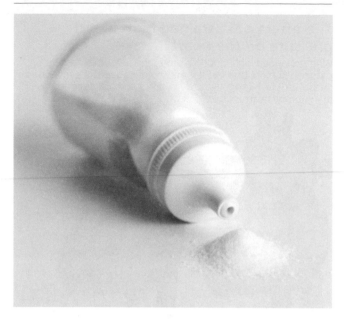

salt intake helps to reduce blood pressure. A high salt intake over many years probably raises blood pressure by raising the sodium content of the smooth muscle cells of the walls of the arterioles. This high sodium content appears to facilitate the entry of calcium into the cells; this in turn causes them to contract and narrow the internal diameter of the arteriole.

There is some evidence that people with an inherited tendency to develop hypertension have a reduced capacity to remove salt from their bodies. There is, however, little evidence that such people consume more salt than anyone else, although they may tend to retain what they do eat.

Evidence from studies
The relationship between salt and hypertension has,

over the years, been controversial mainly because the original research was not carried out carefully enough. However, during the mid-1980s a very reliable international comparative study showed convincingly that there is a close relationship between salt intake and blood pressure when comparing people in 32 different countries. For instance, people who are Japanese, Polish and Portuguese have a high salt intake and a high frequency of raised blood pressure and strokes.

Furthermore, it was found that those populations that have a large amount of salt in their diet are also those populations in which blood pressure rises more with advancing age. By contrast populations in which salt intake is low show only a small rise in blood pressure with advancing age and thus hypertension is relatively less common. As I discuss later in this book, there is now good evidence that reducing the amount of salt in the diet does lower blood pressure.

It is certainly true, however, that there are variations in the way individuals' bodies handle salt and some people are more sensitive to it than others. This is probably true of people with a strong family history of hypertension and it is also evident that older people are more salt sensitive, as are people of African–Caribbean origin.

Children and salt

The relationship between salt intake and the subsequent development of hypertension has recently been confirmed by a reliable study which began by looking at babies who were weaned on to either a low-salt diet or a normal-salt diet. After six months the blood pressure was better (lower) in the low-salt babies. A proportion of these babies has now been followed up for 15 years and their blood pressures were found still to be significantly lower.

If children could be persuaded to consume less salt then we might prevent the development of hypertension in the first place, which means that we should be seriously concerned about the amount of salt in crisps and other snacks that children nowadays consume in large quantities. The food industry is now under pressure from the Food Standards Agency to reduce the salt and fat content of processed and convenience foods, and is starting to respond. A recent study has shown that children who consume large quantities of sugary fizzy drinks also tend to consume more salty snacks.

It is interesting to note that a high salt intake has now been implicated as a cause of stomach cancer, asthma and osteoporosis (bone mineral loss).

Your weight

Overweight people tend to have higher blood pressures than thin people. This is partly because obese people's bodies have to work harder to burn up the excess calories that they consume, partly because they tend to eat more salt than normal, and possibly because fat people have a tendency to be resistant to the hormone insulin, which deals with blood sugar (glucose), and this may be involved in causing hypertension, although it is not yet fully understood.

Although overweight people do appear to have higher blood pressure than people of normal weight, this may in part be related to a tendency for doctors and nurses using blood pressure machines to overestimate their blood pressure. The greater the circumference of the upper arm where the blood pressure cuff is applied, the greater the overestimation of blood pressure. This can partly be overcome if they make sure that they use a larger arm cuff when appropriate.

Body mass index

However, even when allowances have been made for this tendency to overestimate blood pressure, there is still a convincing relationship between body weight and blood pressure. It's not possible to say whether you are overweight just on the basis of how much you actually weigh (because tall people usually weigh more than short people), so instead doctors usually work out what's called the body mass index (BMI). This is calculated by taking your weight in kilograms and dividing it by the square of your height in metres (see box on page 50).

A person who has a body mass index of 30 or more is considered to be obese, whereas if it is between 25 and 30 he or she would be considered to be overweight.

Waist-to-hip ratio

Recent evidence strongly suggests that body mass index is not the best risk factor for the development of cardiovascular disease. Attention is now turning to 'waist/hip ratio'. This implies that, if the waist measurement is increased (as with a paunch or beer belly) in comparison with the hip measurements, there is a greater chance of developing hypertension, diabetes, heart attacks and strokes.

What should you weigh?

- The body mass index (BMI) is a useful measure of healthy weight
- Find out your height in metres and weight in kilograms
- Calculate your BMI like this:

$$BMI = \frac{\text{Your weight (kg)}}{[\text{Your height (metres)} \times \text{Your height (metres)}]}$$

$$\text{e.g. } 24.8 = \frac{70}{[1.68 \times 1.68]}$$

- You are recommended to try to maintain a BMI in the range 18.5–24.9
- The chart below is an easier way of estimating your BMI. Read off your height and your weight. The point where the lines cross in the chart indicates your BMI

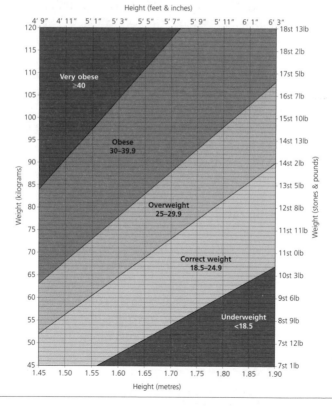

The importance of losing weight

Population surveys have shown that the variation in blood pressure between people in relation to their weight is about one millimetre of mercury (mmHg) per kilogram (or two pounds) in weight. When you put on weight the amount that you gain is a good guide to the amount by which your blood pressure will rise. If you lose weight your blood pressure will fall by an amount that can be predicted using the same formula.

The relationship between body weight and blood pressure is more complex than was originally thought and it may also be related to important effects of certain hormones as well as to the body's capacity to handle salt. From a practical point of view, however, losing weight is a very effective way of reducing your blood pressure.

Alcohol

Alcohol has an effect on blood pressure and, on the whole, the more alcohol you drink the higher your blood pressure, although it is not understood why this is. However, teetotallers do tend to have slightly higher blood pressures than very moderate drinkers. In men this means that one or two glasses of wine per day may have a very slightly protective effect against heart disease. The safe level of drinking in women is about two-thirds that of men, that is one glass per day.

People who drink more than this and also people who abuse alcohol are very likely to have raised blood pressure and have a strong tendency to develop strokes. When such people stop drinking their blood pressure comes down.

Although the relationship between alcohol and blood pressure is now well recognised, surprisingly no

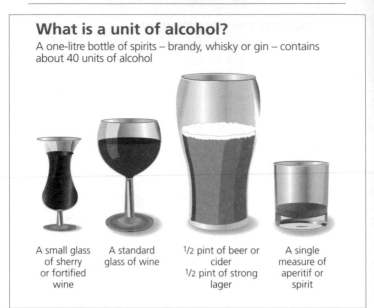

What is a unit of alcohol?

A one-litre bottle of spirits – brandy, whisky or gin – contains about 40 units of alcohol

A small glass of sherry or fortified wine

A standard glass of wine

1/2 pint of beer or cider
1/2 pint of strong lager

A single measure of aperitif or spirit

one has yet discovered a convincing mechanism to explain how this happens. However, from a practical point of view doctors recommend that men should drink no more than 21 units of alcohol per week (equivalent to 10.5 pints of beer or 21 small glasses of wine) and women should drink no more than 14 units per week (equivalent to 7 pints of beer or 14 small glasses of wine). These units should be spread over the week, not drunk all in one session. A better recommendation is that you should consume no more than three alcoholic drinks per day if you are male and two if you are female.

Stress

Stress can put up your blood pressure in the short term but probably does not account for long-term rises in blood pressure. Relaxation techniques may help to improve your quality of life, but probably won't be enough to control true hypertension.

The relationship between stress and blood pressure is confusing and much of the earlier research in this field was not satisfactory by modern standards.

Short-term stress

There is no doubt that acutely stressful stimuli can cause a sharp rise in blood pressure. For example, if you are given some extremely bad or distressing news, your blood pressure may be raised soon afterwards. Similarly, in experimental situations the stress of conducting mental arithmetic in a noisy environment or even sorting out different-sized objects causes a sudden sharp rise in blood pressure.

If going to see a doctor, whether it's your GP or in a hospital clinic, makes you feel anxious and nervous, your blood pressure is likely to go up. For this reason, you should be asked to come back and have it measured again on several occasions if it is slightly raised on your first visit. The idea is that, once you have become more familiar with the environment and the procedure, you will be better able to relax and the reading will then be a more accurate reflection of your blood pressure when you are not under any stress.

Chronic (long-term) stress

Although the effects of this kind of short-term stress on blood pressure are well recognised, there is little evidence that chronic (that is, long-term) stress causes chronic hypertension. Reliable studies have shown no relationship between levels of stress, as assessed by detailed and accurate questioning, and the height of blood pressure. People with very stressful jobs do not have more hypertension or heart disease than people with unstressful jobs. The research in this field has been seriously hampered by the lack of reliable measures of stress so the subject remains somewhat controversial.

There is some evidence that people who have less control over their day-to-day life at work have higher blood pressures than people who can influence their working lives more effectively. Thus manual workers tend to have higher blood pressures than executives or managers. The differences between these groups are, however, also related to differences in lifestyle and diet, and it is difficult to be sure whether they are the result of stress alone.

Potassium

Eating lots of foods that contain potassium – such as fruit and vegetables – is good for keeping blood pressure low. However, people with high-potassium diets often have fairly low salt intake, so it's hard to know whether it's the low salt or the high potassium that is helping. That said, potassium does seem to be beneficial in its own right. There is quite good evidence that people who have a low-potassium diet have higher blood pressure, whereas those who eat a lot of fruit and vegetables have lower blood pressure and a lower incidence of stroke. This makes sense because we know that cells respond to high potassium by getting rid of sodium (in salt).

This effect of potassium intake on blood pressure is small compared with that of salt. However, it is true to say that variations in salt intake between people are also associated with parallel variations in potassium intake. In other words, people who eat

The importance of healthy eating

Eat plenty of fruit and vegetables to improve your general health and well-being.

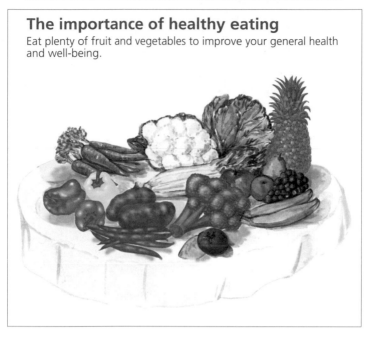

a lot of potassium-rich foods generally eat relatively little salt, whereas salt fans tend to eat fewer fruit and vegetables.

This finding was confirmed in 2006 with the publication of a detailed overview of all of the population studies on fruit and vegetable intake and stroke. This demonstrated that people who consume more than five portions of fruit and/or vegetables each day have a significantly lower stroke incidence than those consuming fewer than three servings per day. Another study, also published in 2006, raised a strong possibility that it is the vegetable protein in pulses and nuts that keeps the blood pressure down, although there may also be an effect related to the higher potassium content.

The effect of diet on blood pressure

This shows the effects of a normal (control) diet and the DASH diet (low in dairy products and animal fats and high in fruit and vegetables) on systolic blood pressure while on a high-, intermediate- and low-salt diet. Changing from an unhealthy to a healthy diet drops the systolic blood pressure by a total of 8.9 mmHg, and is an effect roughly equivalent to that of a single antihypertensive drug.

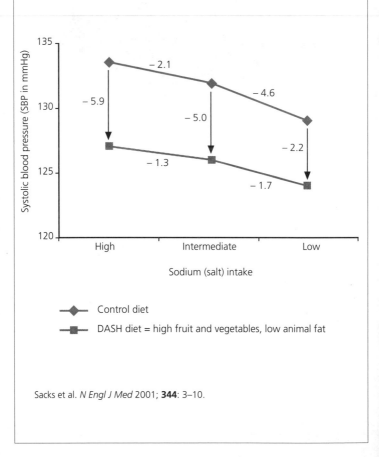

Sacks et al. *N Engl J Med* 2001; **344**: 3–10.

Animal fats

Early studies on the relationship between the intakes of animal fats (mainly in the form of dairy products) were unconvincing. However, a very reliable recent study from America has shown that a reduction in animal fat intake was associated with a significant fall in blood pressure.

The effect of diet on blood pressure

A very well-conducted study in the USA, the Dietary Approaches to Stop Hypertension (DASH) trial, showed convincingly that a reduced animal fat diet and an increased intake of fruit and vegetables both lowered blood pressure in people with normal blood pressure as well as those with hypertension. The two diets when put together had an additive effect on each other. Furthermore there was a further reduction in blood pressure when participants also reduced their salt intake.

Thus changing from an unhealthy to a healthy diet dropped the systolic blood pressure by a total of 8.9 mmHg, and is an effect roughly equivalent to that of a single antihypertensive drug.

It is clear that there are many nutritional factors that influence blood pressure and these are the subject of a major international research project, which was started in 1997. The final results show that almost all of the differences in blood pressure between individuals can be explained by nutritional and lifestyle factors, after taking into account the effects of age.

Exercise

Although your blood pressure rises sharply while you're actually exercising, if you do it regularly you will tend to be healthier and have lower blood pressure than people who don't take any exercise. This is partly because you are more likely to eat healthily, not smoke and not drink excessive alcohol, although exercise also seems to have a direct effect on lowering blood pressure. However, you should aim to take regular, moderate amounts of exercise rather than going in for very vigorous bouts every now and again.

The symptoms of hypertension

The vast majority of people with hypertension have no symptoms. Some people believe that they can feel their blood pressure but, in fact, it is more likely that they are feeling the emotional stress of attending hospital or some recent stressful event in their life. This short-term stress may or may not raise the blood pressure.

The fact that hypertension causes no symptoms means that it is often not diagnosed for many years, by which time the person has subtle evidence of damage to the heart, brain or kidneys. At a later stage, the person may go to the doctor because he or she has started to feel unwell. He or she may, for example, have had a small stroke or have angina (chest pain on exertion), or even have had a heart attack. Someone who has developed heart failure may feel breathless when lying down, whereas kidney failure can be responsible for general tiredness and exhaustion as well as breathlessness.

Don't wait to feel ill before having your blood pressure checked

These are serious problems, which is why you should never wait until you feel ill before having your blood pressure checked. The current opinion is that everyone over the age of 20 should have a routine blood pressure check by their GP. The likelihood is that your reading will be normal or require no action and, if so, you probably need to be re-checked only every three or four years, but some people with borderline pressures may need to be checked more often.

Younger people and children who have obesity or kidney disease or a strong family history of hypertension should also be checked routinely.

How common is hypertension?

Hypertension is more common with advancing age, particularly in populations who have a high salt intake, so age must be taken into account when we consider the prevalence of hypertension.

Premenopausal women (having monthly periods) tend to have lower blood pressure than men of the same age, although the difference between the sexes becomes less apparent over the age of 50 years. This is because, before the menopause, women may be relatively protected from heart disease by the female hormone, oestrogen. Oestrogen levels fall after the menopause and women start to catch up with men in terms of developing heart disease.

Any dividing line between so-called high blood pressure and normal blood pressure must be purely arbitrary. Even if your blood pressure is around the average for the population as a whole, you are at higher risk than someone whose blood pressure is persistently below this level. Thus a blood pressure of 140/80 mmHg carries a slightly worse prognosis (outlook) than blood pressure of 130/70 mmHg.

As explained earlier, the most useful definition of hypertension is therefore that level of blood pressure where treatment is necessary to prevent the individual developing heart disease, stroke and other complications of hypertension. At the present state of knowledge, on the basis of reliable trials of the drug treatment of hypertension compared with dummy (placebo) tablets, we know that treatment is necessary if the blood pressure is consistently 160/100 mmHg or more at all ages.

This threshold is lower in people who are at high risk by virtue of having had a heart attack or a stroke, or if they also have diabetes. In such people, treatment is now recommended if the blood pressure is consistently above 140/85 to 140/90 mmHg.

Around 25 per cent of people have a diastolic blood pressure of 90 mmHg or more, although it is worth stressing that many of them will have a lower reading on re-checking so that no treatment may be necessary. Should the level not fall when your blood pressure is measured again, you may need drug treatment.

If your diastolic pressure is below 90 mmHg, but your systolic pressure is over 160 mmHg, you will be diagnosed as having isolated systolic hypertension (ISH). This condition is vary rare in people under the age of 60 but affects 20 to 30 per cent of those over the age of 80. Recent research has shown that treatment to lower the systolic pressure is very effective at preventing heart attacks and strokes in patients with ISH.

If we take into consideration all types of hypertension affecting people over the age of 60, about 35 to 40 per cent of men and women in the UK need further assessment on the basis of either a raised diastolic or a raised systolic blood pressure. However, this percentage is lower among people whose consumption of salt is below the national average.

Geographical variation

Surveys suggest that between seven and ten million people in the UK have raised blood pressure levels. Socioeconomic factors seem to play a part – people who live in poorer areas are more likely to have hypertension than those who live in more affluent areas. Certainly, heart disease and strokes are more prevalent in the north and north-west of England, in Wales and in Scotland than in the south-east of England, although this also reflects smoking habits.

It must be stressed that many blood pressures are only slightly raised and will be lower on re-checking. Estimates of the number of people with raised blood pressure who require drug treatment vary between 10 and 15 per cent of the adult population. This represents a very small proportion of people aged 20 to 30 years but about half of those over the age of 70.

Hypertension is therefore the most common chronic, non-infective, medical condition in the world. About 50 million people in the USA have blood pressure levels that require treatment and a similar figure is seen in studies from the European Union. The prevalence of hypertension in the UK is higher than in France, Italy, Spain and Greece, and similar to that seen in Sweden and Denmark. In both the UK and the USA, however, hypertension is much more common in people of African origin. The reasons for this are not entirely clear, but it is possible that these people tend to handle the salt in their diet in a different way, such that their bodies retain more of it and this puts their blood pressure up. For more on this, see page 118.

Death rate from CHD by area in the UK

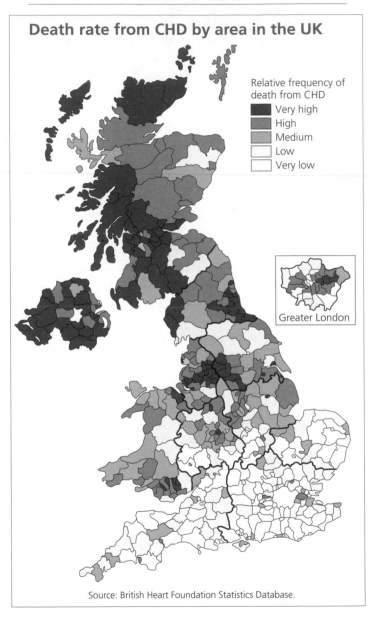

Relative frequency of
death from CHD

- Very high
- High
- Medium
- Low
- Very low

Greater London

Source: British Heart Foundation Statistics Database.

KEY POINTS

■ Hypertension runs in families

■ Hypertension is related to a high salt intake, being overweight and drinking too much alcohol

■ Rarely, high blood pressure is the result of underlying kidney disease or excess hormones

How hypertension is investigated

Why are further tests needed?

People whose blood pressure levels are found to be raised need to have further tests and investigations. There are three main reasons why this might be considered necessary:

1   To check your cholesterol levels: if you have a high blood cholesterol level as well as hypertension, your risk of developing heart disease and strokes (cardiovascular risk) is correspondingly greater, and you will need treatment to bring both blood pressure and cholesterol levels back down to normal.

2   To check for underlying diseases that cause hypertension: occasionally, hypertension may be caused by certain kidney diseases and some extremely rare diseases of the adrenal gland which is situated above the kidney.

3   To check for heart and kidney damage: this may
    occur after prolonged untreated hypertension, so
    blood tests are taken to measure kidney function
    and the size of the heart is estimated by an
    electrocardiogram (ECG). A chest X-ray does not
    give a reliable indication of heart size and is not
    recommended.

Routine tests

All people with raised blood pressure need a simple
urine test; a small blood specimen is taken and an ECG
must be taken. You'll be weighed and, if necessary,
given advice on how to lose weight which is likely to
help reduce your blood pressure.

Routine investigations
Your weight will be measured.

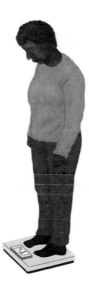

Routine investigations (contd)

Your doctor will examine your chest.

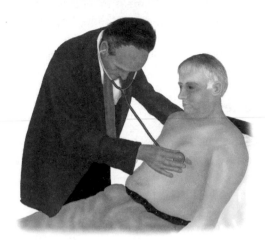

Your doctor will examine your tummy.

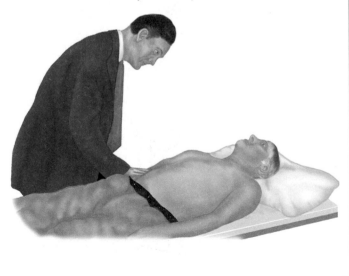

Routine investigations (contd)

Your doctor may examine your ankles for swelling or to check the pulses in your feet.

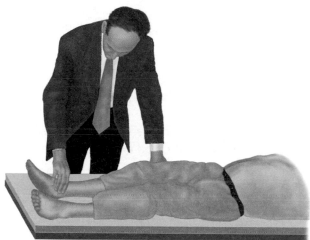

A small blood sample may be taken.

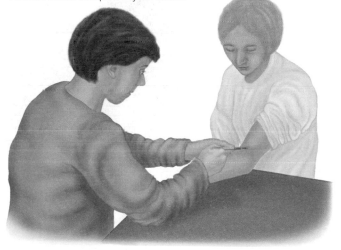

Next your doctor will examine your heart, chest, tummy and the pulses in your legs. This may give some indication as to whether hypertension has affected your heart or kidneys.

The type of heart damage called heart failure results in fluid retention which causes fluid on the lungs that can be heard through a stethoscope. It can also cause an enlarged left side of the heart which the doctor can detect. Kidney damage can be diagnosed only by urine and blood tests.

If your hypertension is very severe, the doctor will probably use an instrument called an ophthalmoscope to look at the back of your eyes (the retina) where it is possible to assess the tiny blood vessels. In mild hypertension these blood vessels show only very minor

Routine investigations (contd)

Your doctor may look at your retina.

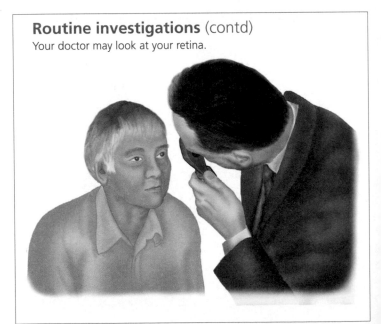

changes, but in a very severe hypertension there may be haemorrhages on the retina and areas of damage that are referred to as 'cotton-wool spots'.

Urine test

After the clinical examination, you'll be asked to produce a small specimen of urine for testing. If sugar is found in the urine, this raises the possibility that you may have diabetes and, if protein is found in the urine, it could mean that you have some form of kidney condition. It is only fairly recently that the serious significance of the presence of protein in the urine has been fully appreciated. It is mandatory that a routine urine test be carried out in all people with any form of hypertension.

Blood test

Blood tests are taken to measure your serum total cholesterol and the amount of HDL (good) cholesterol and to test the function of your kidneys. If the kidney function is normal, the serum creatinine is usually below 120 micromoles/litre (μmol/l). The patient would be considered to have severe renal failure if the serum creatinine is greater than 600 μmol/l. If the kidneys are not working properly, levels of urea and creatinine in the blood start to rise. In addition levels of sodium and potassium in the blood are measured. These are abnormal in people with hypertension whose bodies retain sodium because of the presence of a small benign tumour of the adrenal gland producing the hormone called aldosterone; this condition is called Conn's syndrome.

Electrocardiogram

An ECG gives a recording of the electrical activity of the heart. It has a dual purpose. First, it can give an indirect index of the size of the heart. When the blood pressure is very high, the heart enlarges in order to cope with increased load and this leads to increased voltages on the ECG. This is called left ventricular hypertrophy (or LVH) and is very important. When someone is found to have LVH, their need for treatment to lower their blood

Exercise ECG

Patients with suspected disease of the coronary artery and high blood pressure may undergo an exercise ECG while walking on a treadmill. This is conducted under close medical supervision. The ECG during exercise may well show changes of ischaemia or poor perfusion of the wall of the heart that are not present at rest.

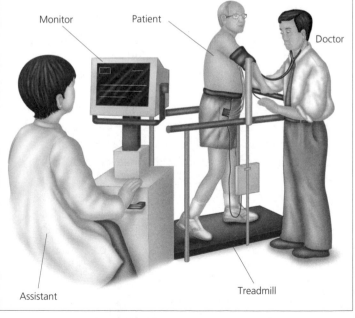

Monitor

Patient

Doctor

Assistant

Treadmill

pressure becomes more urgent because it indicates that the heart muscle is under significant strain trying to cope with the effort of pumping blood out round the body at increased pressure.

The second reason for doing an ECG is because it may show changes suggestive of narrowing or blockage of the coronary arteries, which supply the heart muscle. This process is called 'ischaemia' and is seen in some people who experience angina (chest pain) on exertion. Even though you may never have had symptoms of angina and have no reason to think that you've ever had a heart attack, you may nevertheless show signs of ischaemic changes and these are important.

Further tests

These are the routine investigations that are needed by everyone with hypertension. You will require the more detailed investigations only if your hypertension is severe enough or if your doctor suspects that you have some underlying condition that is responsible for your blood pressure problems.

Up to five per cent of people with hypertension are found to have underlying medical conditions that cause their pressure to be high. These are diseases of the kidney and of the adrenal gland. In this situation, you will probably be referred to a specialist clinic in your local hospital. A further three or four per cent of people have very severe hypertension that needs more detailed investigation and care by a specialist in high blood pressure.

The vast majority of people with hypertension do not and should not attend hospital for any reason at all and can be cared for by their GP. There will be marked variations in the proportion of patients referred to hospital clinics, depending on the availability of local services and specialist blood pressure doctors. Whether you have to attend a hospital clinic will depend on your individual GP's policy in such cases. Some may refer a large number of their patients to be seen only once or twice for a full assessment in hospital and then look after them themselves, whereas others refer only the very difficult cases to a hospital specialist.

Suspicion of there being some underlying cause for the hypertension would be based on the presence of protein in the urine or abnormal routine blood test results, showing evidence of impairment of kidney function. In addition, if levels of potassium in the blood are found to be low, this raises the possibility that there may be an underlying condition of the adrenal glands (Conn's syndrome).

You will also be referred to a hospital clinic if your blood pressure varies greatly from minute to minute or hour to hour or even day to day. There is an extremely rare condition called phaeochromocytoma which is caused by the intermittent secretion of large quantities of adrenaline and noradrenaline by a tumour of the adrenal gland. Most patients with this condition have symptoms from attacks of a very fast pulse rate (palpitations) and headaches

When you do go to a clinic, you may have to undergo a repeat of some of the blood tests already done by your GP merely to confirm abnormalities. If there is a suspicion that you may have Conn's syndrome, in which the hypertension is the result of excess of a hormone called aldosterone, the hospital doctor may opt to measure this in your blood.

Ultrasound

Ultrasound investigation of the kidneys.

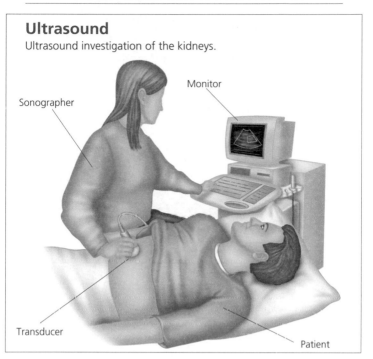

Monitor

Sonographer

Transducer

Patient

Kidney ultrasound

To exclude any form of kidney disease, it is usual to do an ultrasound scan to investigate the size and shape of the kidneys. This test is increasingly becoming a routine investigation for severely hypertensive people because it is safe and causes no discomfort.

24-hour urine tests

You may also be asked to provide a 24-hour collection of urine so that your body's 24-hour output of adrenaline and noradrenaline can be measured (don't worry, the clinic will provide the bottles). Raised levels could indicate that you have a phaeochromocytoma (see above).

Echocardiography

An instrument called a transducer, which produces a beam of sound, is held against the chest. A picture of the heart is created by the reflected sound beams.

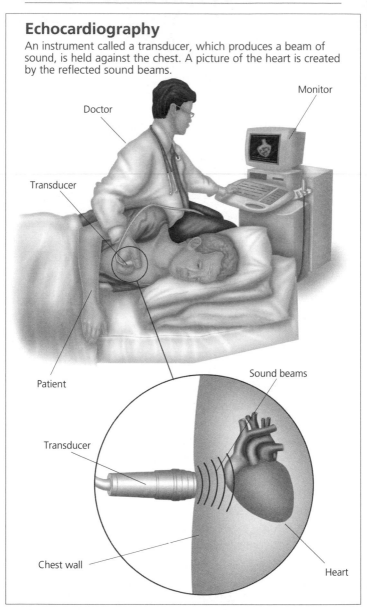

Monitor

Doctor

Transducer

Patient

Sound beams

Transducer

Chest wall

Heart

Echocardiogram

The clinic doctor may also measure your heart size by means of an echocardiogram, which is a type of ultrasound heart scan. The echocardiogram provides a more sensitive screening test for enlargement of the heart than the ECG. If this test does show enlargement, then an antihypertensive drug is absolutely essential.

Tailoring treatments

Very often, people are referred to a hospital clinic because their blood pressure is proving a little resistant to treatment and the hospital doctor may therefore opt to alter drug combinations and formulations in order to obtain better blood pressure control.

Once your blood pressure is under control and things are sorted out you will normally be discharged from the care of the clinic back to your GP, and have to go back to the hospital only if problems arise. Once blood pressure is controlled, you should visit your practice nurse every three months and your family doctor about once a year for routine checks.

KEY POINTS

- All people diagnosed as hypertensive should have a spot urine check, a single blood test and an ECG

- Only a minority of patients need referral to specialist clinics for hypertension for further investigation

Treatment without drugs

Importance of diet and lifestyle

This is sometimes called 'non-pharmacological' blood pressure reduction and it has been shown to work. It generally involves relatively straightforward changes to your diet and lifestyle which you can make with advice from your GP, although you may find some harder to do than others. Nevertheless, it really is worth making a big effort because, if you are successful, your blood pressure may return to normal without the need for drug treatment.

Reducing salt intake

Your GP will almost certainly advise you to reduce the amount of salt that you consume. In the UK, the average salt intake in men is about 10 grams per day and in women it is about six to seven grams per day. However, a very large number of people consume about half this amount and they have lower blood pressures. Only about one gram of daily salt intake is added to food when it's on the table or during cooking. The rest comes mostly in processed foods, including burgers, meat pies, sausages, cheeses, salted snacks, tinned foods (such as vegetables), breakfast cereals and bread.

You can help cut your intake by never adding salt to your food at the table or when cooking. Try to make more use of fresh meat and fresh fruit and vegetables, and only eat processed foods as the exception rather than the rule. All herbs and spices can be used safely to flavour foods in place of salt when cooking.

Making changes

Adjusting to a low-salt diet can be a little difficult at first but you will probably find that, if you can consistently keep your salt intake down, then after about a month or so you actually prefer your food with less salt.

If you were then to go back to your old eating habits, you would find that your food tastes too salty and that you have become 'converted'.

It's much the same process as happens to people who stop adding large quantities of sugar to their tea or coffee. Once they get used to drinking unsweetened tea or coffee, they often find that adding even a tiny amount of sugar makes it taste so repulsive that they would rather drink water. The same thing can happen when changing from a high-salt to a low-salt diet.

Salt and the food industry

Sadly, the food industry has responded to the salt/blood pressure problem only in a limited manner. Salt was once a useful preservative but modern food technology and refrigeration mean that the salt content of processed foods can be reduced. Unfortunately, many people have now become 'hooked' on salty foods.

There has been some irresponsible propaganda by some representatives of the food industry in which they have suggested that there is no relationship between salt and blood pressure, and that all the experts who have done research in this field are wrong.

Experts do not necessarily advocate a drastic reduction in salt intake; they advocate bringing it down to the same level as that in the diets of a great many people who tend to prefer good quality food without preservatives or additives.

There is some evidence that the lower blood pressures in people in senior positions in executive and managerial jobs are related to their lower salt intake, as well as to the fact that fewer of them are overweight.

Salt substitutes

There are several salt substitutes now available from chemist shops. These contain less sodium chloride and more potassium chloride. Although, in an ideal world, no one should need to add crystals of any chemical substance to their food, if you really can't tolerate food with a low-salt content you can use the salt substitutes instead, but only if your kidney function has been shown to be normal.

Don't forget, though, that sea salt, rock salt and 'natural' salt are still salt (that is, sodium chloride) and so are not salt substitutes. You need to use salt substitutes with care if you are taking a 'potassium-sparing' drug such as the water pills spironolactone or amiloride or the angiotensin-converting enzyme (ACE) inhibitors or the angiotensin receptor blockers (ARBs) and if your kidneys are not functioning well, as you may have high potassium levels anyway. If in doubt, ask your GP's advice.

Weight control

As was pointed out earlier, for every kilogram (two pounds) of weight that you lose your blood pressure will fall by about one millimetre of mercury. So, if it is only slightly elevated, say around 165/95 mmHg, it may go down to normal if you manage to lose a stone in weight. There is reliable evidence from clinical trials to show that losing weight does lower blood pressure. It's not easy to do, however, unless you have proper advice and strong motivation, and your diet should take account of the need to cut your salt intake as well.

Research indicates that, if you are overweight, you are likely to lose more if you're referred to a dietician or nutritionist than if you're simply told to lose weight by your doctor. You also have a better chance of reaching your target weight if you increase the amount of exercise that you take and cut down the amount of alcohol that you drink, if appropriate.

Almost all medical authorities in all specialities agree that we should all adopt 'the prudent diet' with:

- less salt

- less animal fat

- more fish

- more fruit and vegetables.

This diet is associated with protection from many diseases, including cancer.

Sensible alcohol consumption

There is good evidence that drinking only moderate amounts of alcohol lowers blood pressure and you probably don't need to give it up altogether. The Royal Colleges of Physicians, Psychiatrists and General Practitioners in the UK recommend a maximum intake of 21 units of alcohol per week for men and 14 units for women. Avoid binge drinking because it can cause strokes. There is some recent evidence that older people are more prone to alcohol-induced damage. It is likely therefore that older people should be advised to drink less than the 21 and 14 units mentioned above.

It may be the case that having one to two drinks every day may be associated with lower levels of heart disease. However, more than four drinks per day does appear to be associated with increased risk of hypertension and stroke, as well as having damaging effects on the liver, the nervous system and the quality of life.

Taking exercise

Research has proved a clear association between taking more exercise and a fall in blood pressure. The mechanisms are not entirely certain and may in part be related to dietary changes that people often make at the same time as they begin exercising regularly. If you have hypertension, however, you need to use your common sense when deciding on your exercise programme. For example, an overweight middle-aged man with severe hypertension who has never taken any exercise would be unwise to take up vigorous exercise that leaves him feeling exhausted. It is much better to opt for a graded programme of gradually increasing exercise.

Start by using stairs rather than a lift or escalator whenever you have to climb only two or three flights, and try walking to a more distant car park or bus stop on the way to and from work or the shops. Any form of sport is fine provided that you don't exhaust yourself, but you need to put in sufficient effort to cause a small rise in your pulse rate and make you feel that you are sweating a bit.

Potassium supplements

Although there is evidence that increasing the amount of potassium in the diet lowers your blood pressure, you should not take supplements in the form of potassium salts or tablets. Instead, you should increase the amount of potassium in your diet by eating more fresh fruit and vegetables and cutting your salt intake from processed foods at the same time.

Stress counselling

As explained earlier, there is little evidence that chronic stress causes high blood pressure. However, there are many people with hypertension who are immensely stressed for a multitude of reasons, as a result of personal problems, anxieties at work or the development of anxiety states for which no obvious cause can be found.

If this applies to you, stress counselling and, in extreme cases, psychiatric treatment may help to reduce your stress and your blood pressure may come down at the same time. Otherwise, there is no reason to believe that most people with hypertension will derive any benefit from stress counselling, relaxation therapies, yoga, biofeedback or other related techniques.

What you may find is that, after stress counselling, you are more able to relax when you see your doctor, but this type of treatment for stress does not appear to affect the continuous 24-hour home blood pressure readings that are obtained by electronic blood pressure monitors.

This is a controversial area, but the current view is that the role of stress counselling and the like in the management of hypertension has, to date, been over- rather than understated.

Complementary therapies

A great many complementary and so-called 'natural' products have been tried out in the management of people with raised blood pressure.

Two large and very reliable studies show that antioxidant vitamins have no effect on blood pressure or cardiovascular risk, and these are emphatically not recommended.

Recently, a yoghurt-type product containing sour milk has been shown to have a trivial effect on blood pressure. However, for this to be effective on a long-term basis, you would need to consume two containers of this yoghurt every day for 20 to 30 years and so this regimen is also not recommended.

There is some evidence that garlic may have a small effect on blood pressure. Most of the garlic that we consume is in foods that are of a higher standard and it may well be that it is these other contents of the foods that are beneficial. It is, however, true that garlic is not harmful.

KEY POINTS

- Relatively straightforward changes to your diet and lifestyle can reduce your blood pressure and remove the need for drug treatment

- There is good evidence that reducing the amount of salt in the diet does reduce blood pressure

- If you are overweight, reducing your weight will lower your blood pressure

- Research has proved a clear association between taking regular exercise and a fall in blood pressure

Drug treatment

The development of drug treatment

Until the 1950s there was almost nothing that doctors could do to reduce blood pressure. People with severe hypertension became unwell with strokes, heart and kidney failure, and their doctors could only stand helplessly by.

During the late 1950s and early 1960s, antihypertensive drugs became available that did lower blood pressure and did save lives. Many of these early drugs, which are no longer used, were, however, associated with severe side effects and their use was justified only in patients with a very poor outlook.

During the 1970s drugs with fewer and less dramatic side effects became available and these could therefore be given to people with milder hypertension who were at a lower cardiovascular risk.

A large number of well-conducted trials were performed in which active treatment was compared with placebo (dummy) tablets. All of these trials were discontinued the moment it could be shown that people taking the active treatment developed fewer heart attacks and strokes than those receiving placebo.

Pooling the results of all these trials, we now know that antihypertensive drug therapy for all grades of hypertension brings about a 35 to 40 per cent reduction of strokes and a 20 to 25 per cent reduction in coronary heart disease.

People with hypertension may of course develop heart attacks as a result of other factors, for example, cigarette smoking or having high blood cholesterol levels. It is now, however, true to say that the complications of hypertension should be avoidable if blood pressure can be controlled.

The development of antihypertensive drugs with minimal side effects and their immense benefits in terms of prevention of heart attacks and strokes has been one of the biggest advances in medical care since World War II. It is at least comparable with the revolution that was achieved with the development of effective antibiotics.

Blood pressure-lowering drugs have also been shown to be effective in reducing or preventing kidney damage in people with diabetes with or without concurrent hypertension, and more recently some drugs have been shown to prevent damage to the retinas of people with diabetes.

Furthermore, treatment with certain antihypertensive agents can reduce the likelihood of people who have had heart attacks from having a second one or developing heart failure.

Treating elderly people
Everyone whose blood pressure consistently exceeds 160/100 mmHg should take antihypertensive drugs, whatever their age.

Antihypertensive drug treatment is particularly effective in people aged 60 to 80 years who, if not given medication of this kind, face a high risk of having a stroke. Older people often worry that they may suffer a stroke, but they can be reassured that drug treatment can largely prevent this happening, which is an excellent reason to keep taking the tablets as prescribed.

In 2008 a drug trial of the treatment of patients aged over 80 years was published (see page 135). It was called the Hypertension in the Very Elderly Trial (HYVET). Compared with placebo (dummy tablets), antihypertensive drug therapy led to a 30 per cent reduction in strokes, a 64 per cent reduction in heart failure and a 21 per cent reduction in deaths from all causes. It is unlikely that there will be any more long-term outcome trials comparing treatment with no treatment. They are no longer ethically justifiable. The next generation of trials will probably be designed to compare different types of active treatment.

Controlling blood pressure

All drugs that lower blood pressure are roughly equally effective. They drop the systolic pressure by about 10 mmHg and the diastolic pressure by 5 mmHg. Different people respond to them in different ways: for example, older people respond better to some drugs than to others as do people of African–Caribbean origin.

It is worth bearing in mind that much the same falls in blood pressure levels can be achieved by someone who sticks rigorously to advice on restricting salt intake, losing weight and drinking only moderate amounts of alcohol as can be achieved by any single antihypertensive drug.

If you are on drug therapy, you should also remember that the effect of some drugs is greater if you reduce your salt consumption while taking them, so it's worth making the necessary effort to cut down your salt intake.

Using multiple treatments

One tablet a day will be enough to control blood pressure in only around one-quarter of people who are on antihypertensive drug therapy. Most of the rest require double therapy with two different drugs and about 25 per cent of people require triple therapy (that is, three different drugs) to control their blood pressure.

Fortunately, even if you need triple therapy, this usually means taking only three tablets daily. Almost all these can be taken together, either in the morning or in the evening. The older types of drugs, which had to be taken two or three times daily, are now regarded as obsolete. This is good news because the more times you need to take your tablets each day, the more likely you are to forget them sometimes.

Blood pressure that is hard to control

If you are one of the small minority of people whose blood pressure proves very difficult to control you will probably be referred to a specialist and there are a few people whose blood pressure is almost impossible to control. This is probably because they didn't begin taking antihypertensive treatment until a late stage of the disease process, so that the structural changes to the small arterioles are so far advanced that the drugs don't work very well.

It is becoming increasingly clear that many people with apparently uncontrollable hypertension do have a major white coat effect; 24-hour ABPM may reveal that pressures are uncontrolled only when measured in the clinic. Once the patient leaves the clinic ABPM may reveal that the blood pressure is in fact well controlled. This is another reason why guidelines increasingly emphasise the importance of home monitoring.

It must be stressed, however, that most people with hypertension have only mildly raised blood pressure, which is relatively easily controlled and, if you are in this category, you can be cared for perfectly well by your GP and the practice nurse.

A long-term treatment

Many people have the mistaken idea that they will need to take drugs to lower their blood pressure only for a short while, rather like taking a short course of antibiotics, and then they can forget the whole thing. This is an extremely dangerous misunderstanding and, if you give up taking the tablets, your risk of a heart attack or stroke will be greatly increased.

With very few exceptions, antihypertensive treatment needs to be taken for the rest of your life. As you get older, the risk of a stroke increases and so the benefit of treatment is correspondingly greater. If you stop taking the drugs and your blood pressure stays down, it is necessary to question whether you ever really had hypertension in the first place, or whether your treatment was started on the basis of a single raised blood pressure reading taken when you were under stress, just because you were having it measured in an unfamiliar environment. In reality, the chances of anyone with genuine hypertension being able to stop antihypertensive tablets are small.

Changing your lifestyle

However, if your hypertension was only mild in the first place and if you needed no more than one tablet a day to control it, then, if you change to a low-salt, low-fat diet and consume at least five portions of vegetables or fruit per day, and also lose weight, cut down on alcohol and take more exercise, you may be able to come off drug treatment.

Even so, about half the people who do manage to do this will need to re-start therapy at some stage. If your doctor does agree that you should stop treatment, he or she will need to see you regularly for check-ups, at first monthly and thereafter three-monthly. It is very likely that your blood pressure will eventually go up again and you will need to go back on the tablets.

Anyone who needs double therapy (two different drugs) to control their blood pressure is extremely unlikely ever to be able to come off therapy altogether. There is, however, some evidence that people whose blood pressure was initially difficult to control, and who therefore needed triple or quadruple therapy, may develop easier blood pressure control as the years go by, and so be able to manage on fewer drugs.

Stopping treatment

Like many people who have been prescribed antihypertensive drugs, you may be tempted to stop taking them or actually do so without going back to your doctor. It's all too easy to convince yourself that you don't really need them because you're feeling well and have no symptoms. The chances are that, if you do this, you may one day end up in the accident and emergency department of your local hospital, because you have developed one of the complications of hypertension, such as a heart attack or stroke.

Alternatively, you may eventually go back to your doctor with very high blood pressure that is extremely difficult to control, so you then need to take three, four or even five drugs. You can avoid this happening to you if you continue to take the treatment that's been prescribed and attend your doctor's surgery regularly for check-ups.

Monitoring your condition and treatment

Once your hypertension has been assessed by your doctor and been brought under control by treatment, you will probably need to have your blood pressure checked only about four times a year. It is important to go back for such checks to make sure that your blood pressure is under control and, increasingly, your appointments are likely to be with a specially trained practice nurse rather than the doctor.

From time to time, you may need to have other tests besides blood pressure measurement – such as blood tests to check your kidney function or, occasionally, an ECG. Your serum cholesterol levels should also be monitored because high blood cholesterol, like high blood pressure, is an important risk factor for heart disease and cholesterol-lowering treatment also saves lives.

Antihypertensive drugs

There is now a wide choice of blood pressure-lowering drugs. This means that your doctor is able to tailor the treatment to suit your individual needs. It is important for you to know the names of the drugs that you are taking, how they work and their possible side

Controlling hypertension

Regular monitoring of your condition and review of your treatment will ensure that your blood pressure is under the best possible control.

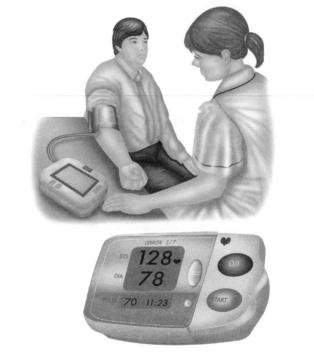

effects. With improvements in drug development, it is becoming increasingly possible to minimise side effects or even avoid them altogether.

The next section of this book describes the currently available drugs. You need to bear in mind that there are usually many different drugs within each of the classes described here and there are minor individual variations between them.

Prescription medication

You may be prescribed medication to help control hypertension.

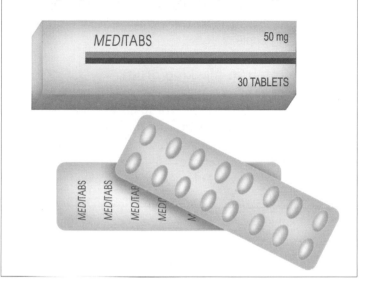

It is a bit confusing, but all drugs have two names. The most prominent name on the box is the proprietary or trade name (for example, Istin, Zestril, Cozaar), but this can vary if several drug companies market the same drug. The small print name is the generic or chemical name (for example, amlodipine, lisinopril, losartan) and gives an idea of which class the drug is in. It is best to use the generic name even if it does seem a bit long at times.

There are three main classes of blood pressure-lowering drugs currently in common use. These are:

1 The angiotensin-blocking drugs
2 The calcium channel-blocking (CCB) drugs
3 The diuretics.

There are other classes of antihypertensive drugs that are still occasionally used in special circumstances. All classes are described in this section but the three listed above are the mainstay of treatment in the vast majority of people.

The angiotensin-blocking drugs

These drugs all block the generation of the hormone, angiotensin II. This hormone constricts the small blood vessels called arterioles and thus increases the resistance to blood flow. As a result of this the blood pressure in the larger arteries rises and hypertension develops. Three classes of angiotensin-blocking drugs are available:

1   The angiotensin-converting enzyme (ACE) inhibitors
2   The angiotensin receptor blockers (ARBs)
3   The direct renin inhibitors (DRIs).

The ACE inhibitors

The first ACE inhibitor, captopril, was introduced in the late 1970s. It is a short-acting drug that has to be taken at least twice daily so it is hardly used nowadays. The commonly used ACE inhibitors are lisinopril, perindopril and ramipril. Many

ACE inhibitors

- Enalapril
- Fosinopril
- Imidapril
- Lisinopril
- Perindopril
- Quinapril
- Ramipril
- Trandolapril

long-term outcome trials have shown that the ACE inhibitors reduce blood pressure and prevent heart attacks and strokes. In addition they reduce or delay the deterioration of kidney function which occurs in people with diabetes and people with primary kidney disease (nephritis). They also delay diabetic eye disease.

The ACE inhibitors have also been shown to increase survival in people with heart failure and those recovering from a heart attack. These beneficial effects on the kidneys, the eyes and the heart appear to be unrelated to the blood pressure-lowering effects because they are seen in people whose blood pressure was not raised

It has become clear therefore that the introduction of the ACE inhibitors was a major breakthrough in the history of hypertension and that is why so many people are being treated with them. The only problem was the side effects.

The ACE inhibitors have two important side effects. One, acute or recurrent angio-oedema, can very rarely be life threatening. The other side effect, a dry cough, can be irritating but is not serious. The angio-oedema is mercifully very rare (1 in 5,000 people) but is seen a bit more often in people of African origin. It causes swelling of the lips and tongue with constriction of the throat. It is commonly intermittent as it comes and goes. If you are receiving an ACE inhibitor and you notice swelling of your lips and tongue, you must stop taking it immediately and make an urgent appointment to see your doctor. You must not be given any ACE inhibitor ever again. There are safer alternatives available (see below).

The dry irritating cough that occurs in about 20 per cent of people receiving an ACE inhibitor is not serious and may be very mild. Indeed you may not realise that you have the cough until someone asks you if you have a cough. Sometimes the cough is so mild that it may not bother you at all, but it may bother your partner as the cough is worse at night.

Despite the two side effects listed above, the ACE inhibitors are remarkably safe and very well

How ACE inhibitors and ARBs work

Angiotensin-converting enzyme (ACE) inhibitors block the activation of the hormone angiotensin II. Angiotensin II is involved in constricting blood vessels. ACE inhibitors therefore open up the blood vessels, lowering blood pressure.

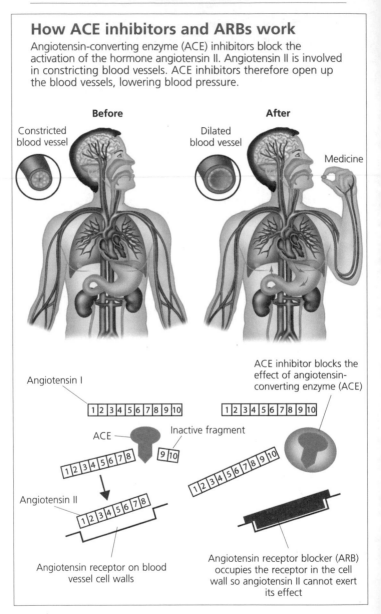

Before

Constricted blood vessel

After

Dilated blood vessel

Medicine

Angiotensin I

ACE   Inactive fragment

Angiotensin II

Angiotensin receptor on blood vessel cell walls

ACE inhibitor blocks the effect of angiotensin-converting enzyme (ACE)

Angiotensin receptor blocker (ARB) occupies the receptor in the cell wall so angiotensin II cannot exert its effect tolerated. It is usual to start at a low dose (for example, lisinopril 5 mg) and increase to the full dose (lisinopril 20 mg) over the period of a few weeks. They should particularly be introduced gradually in people with kidney damage or heart failure.

The angiotensin receptor blockers (ARBs)

The first ARB, losartan, was introduced in 1995. It soon became clear that this agent and its competitors (for example, valsartan, irbesartan, candesartan) did not cause the side effects of cough or angio-oedema that are

Angiotensin receptor blockers

- Candesartan
- Eprosartan
- Irbesartan
- Losartan
- Olmesartan
- Telmisartan
- Valsartan

seen with the ACE inhibitors. Indeed no consistent side effects of the ARBs have been identified. The ARBs are as effective as other agents at reducing blood pressure, and long-term outcome trials show that they are as effective as the ACE inhibitors at reducing heart attacks and strokes. Furthermore, they also reduce the death rate in people who have had a heart attack or heart failure. They also reduce diabetic and non-diabetic kidney damage. There is a body of opinion that the ARBs should replace the ACE inhibitors in routine clinical practice.

Direct renin inhibitors (DRIs)

The only DRI available in the UK is aliskiren, which was introduced in 2005. It is as effective as other angiotensin-blocking drugs at lowering blood pressure and has remarkably few side effects. However, as yet there are no long-term studies to show whether aliskiren reduces heart attacks, strokes, heart failure and renal damage. There is no reason to think that aliskiren will not be shown to be beneficial in these respects. Currently aliskiren should only be given to patients who cannot tolerate an ACE inhibitor or an ARB.

Both the ACE inhibitors and the ARBs are about half as effective at lowering blood pressure in older patients and those of African origin, when compared with the calcium channel blockers and the diuretics. This is not an unexpected finding because it has long been known that these groups of patients have a less active renin–angiotensin system. They do, however, appear to be effective at reducing or delaying renal damage in diabetic and non-diabetic kidney disease in all ages and all ethnic groups. This strongly suggests that the beneficial effects of these drugs on the kidney are unrelated to their blood pressure-lowering actions.

It is for this reason that, in uncomplicated hypertension, the angiotensin-blocking drugs are only recommended as first-line drugs in younger patients and patients of non-African origin.

Calcium channel blockers (CCBs)

These agents were introduced in the early 1980s. They work by blocking the action of calcium in the smooth muscle cells of the wall of the arterioles. It is thought that constriction of the smooth muscle, caused in part by calcium, narrows these blood vessels which causes hypertension to develop.

Calcium channel blockers

- Amlodipine
- Diltiazem
- Felodipine
- Isradipine
- Lacidipine
- Lercanidipine
- Nicardipine
- Nifedipine
- Nisoldipine
- Verapamil

Blocking the action of calcium opens up the blood vessels which results in a fall in blood pressure. The

How calcium channel blockers work

When calcium enters muscle cells they contract. Calcium channel blockers restrict the amount of calcium able to enter cells and so inhibit the contraction of the muscles that line the walls of blood vessels. As a result the blood vessels dilate (open up), reducing blood pressure.

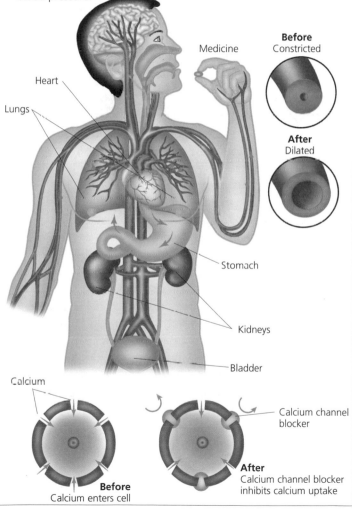

Medicine

Before
Constricted

After
Dilated

Heart

Lungs

Stomach

Kidneys

Bladder

Calcium

Calcium channel blocker

Before
Calcium enters cell

After
Calcium channel blocker inhibits calcium uptake

CCBs are as effective as other agents at lowering blood pressure in all ethnic groups and all ages. They are recommended first-line drugs in older patients and in people of African origin.

The CCBs are sometimes referred to as calcium blockers, calcium antagonists or calcium entry blockers.

There are two classes of CCB:

1   The dihydropyridine (DHP) CCBs
2   The non-dihydropyridine (non-DHP) CCBs.

The DHP CCBs

The first DHP CCB was nifedipine. In its early liquid formulation in a gelatine capsule it was not well tolerated. Once the capsule dissolved in the stomach the active drug was released and absorbed into the bloodstream suddenly. This caused thumping headaches, flushing and an over-rapid fall in blood pressure. When nifedipine became available in tablet form (nifedipine retard), these side effects became less of a problem and now, with a long-acting (LA) tablet formulation, flushing and headache are hardly ever encountered.

The other important side effect of the DHP CCBs is ankle swelling. This swelling is not due to fluid retention, as occurs in congestive heart failure, but is due to tissue (intracellular) fluids leaking into the gaps between the cells. The ankle swelling is not serious or dangerous but it can be very unsightly. It may be more common in women than in men. This side effect is fairly uncommon with the modern LA form of nifedipine.

Amlodipine is a much used DHP CCB. It takes five days to reach its full effect and when stopped it takes as long to wear off. Headaches, flushing and ankle swelling are very rare when this drug is used in the lower dose of five milligrams daily; however, with 10 mg (the top dose) ankle swelling occurs in up to 50 per cent of patients.

When amlodipine is used in combination with an angiotensin-blocking drug, there is good evidence of synergy, that is the two drugs together are more than twice as effective at blood pressure lowering than when either is used alone. There is evidence that the ARB, valsartan, reduces the ankle swelling caused by amlodipine.

Both nifedipine and amlodipine have been evaluated in long-term outcome studies and have been shown to reduce heart attacks and strokes.

The non-DHP CCBs

These are verapamil and diltiazem but they have entirely different chemical structures and also differ from the DHP CCBs. This means that the DHP CCB side effect of ankle swelling almost never occurs. The main side effect of verapamil is constipation. This is not troublesome in most patients but they should be advised to take some form of laxative if constipation is a problem. Only very rarely does this drug have to be abandoned because of this side effect.

Both verapamil and diltiazem are commonly used in patients with heart disease who have no evidence of hypertension.

Both these drugs have been shown to reduce mortality in patients who have survived a heart attack.

Diuretics

The thiazide-type diuretics were introduced in the 1950s and were for many years the mainstay of antihypertensive therapy and have had a lot to do with the reduction of heart attacks and strokes in hypertensive patients over many years. Now with newer and highly effective drugs, the thiazides are declining in use. They are now recommended as third-line agents to be used when the combination of an angiotensin-blocking drug and a calcium channel blocker is insufficient to control the blood pressure. Their main mode of action is to stimulate the kidneys to produce more urine. This leads to a small reduction in the total blood volume and thus a reduction in the pressure in the blood vessels. It is for this reason that diuretics are commonly called 'water pills'. The diuretics also have a direct effect on blood vessels, reducing constriction in the arterioles, which also helps to reduce pressure.

There are three classes of diuretics:

1   The thiazides
2   The thiazide-like diuretics
3   The potassium-retaining diuretics.

The thiazides

The most commonly used thiazide in the UK is bendroflumethiazide (previously bendrofluazide). Given in the low dose of 2.5 mg daily it is effective at lowering blood pressure and preventing heart attacks and strokes. It is also by far the cheapest blood pressure-lowering agent, costing less than 50 pence per month. The main problem with the thiazides is their many effects on body chemistry. They work by making the kidneys remove more salt and water from the body, but occasionally the salt loss can become extreme, causing life-threatening salt deficiency. The

Thiazide diuretics

- Bendroflumethiazide
- Cyclopenthiazide
- Hydrochlorothiazide
- Hydroflumethiazide

How thiazide diuretics work

This class of drugs opens up blood vessels, creating more space for a given volume of blood, so the pressure in the system drops. They also force the kidneys to excrete water and salt, reducing the volume of blood in circulation and therefore the blood pressure.

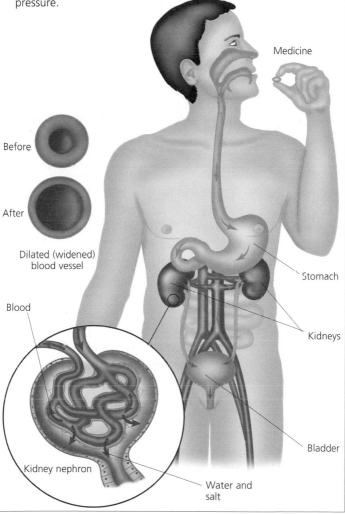

Medicine

Before

After

Dilated (widened) blood vessel

Blood

Stomach

Kidneys

Kidney nephron

Bladder

Water and salt

thiazides also make the kidneys reduce the potassium content of the body and this may have adverse effects on the heart rhythm. In addition, the thiazides cause retention of uric acid, the substance that causes gout, and thiazides can cause a reduction of tolerance to sugar, which can on some occasions actually precipitate the onset of type 2 diabetes. Finally, thiazides can cause men to be unable to obtain or sustain an erection.

Given this long list of side effects it may seem surprising that the thiazides remain so popular. The reason for their continued use is that they were the first antihypertensive drug that was not intolerable. All the predecessors had awful side effects. Furthermore, thiazides definitely save lives; they are highly effective and not expensive. Also the metabolic side effects described above can be minimised if low doses are used.

The thiazide diuretic, hydrochlorothiazide (HCTZ), is not available on its own in the UK. However, it is used in several fixed-dose, two-drug combination pills which include an angiotensin-blocking drug. Examples of these products are lisinopril/HCTZ, losartan/HCTZ and valsartan/HCTZ.

Thiazide-like diuretics

These are chlortalidone (previously chlorthalidone) and indapamide. Both these agents have been shown to reduce heart attacks and strokes. Chlortalidone is particularly popular in the USA, where most of the research has been conducted. It is possible that both these drugs have fewer side effects than bendroflumethiazide. However, it is also possible that the lower incidence of side effects is simply due to the use of lower doses of these agents.

The thiazides and the thiazide-like diuretics are very useful when added to an angiotensin-blocking drug (or a beta blocker – see below). By contrast their use in combination with a CCB is not very effective at lowering blood pressure.

The potassium-retaining diuretics

These are spironolactone and amiloride. They were originally used only in combination to counter the potassium-losing effects of the thiazide diuretics. When used alone they are not very effective and until recently were not much used.

Spironolactone technically speaking is a non-selective aldosterone receptor antagonist (ARA). Aldosterone is a hormone secreted by the adrenal glands, which raised blood pressure by causing salt and water retention. Spironolactone effectively blocks this effect. This drug has, however, been the source of increased interest recently. There is now good trial evidence that spironolactone reduces the death rate in patients with severe heart failure, usually after a heart attack. Most of these patients were receiving an angiotensin-blocking drug as well. These findings led some hypertension specialists to wonder whether spironolactone in low dose might be useful as a fourth-line agent in patients with resistant hypertension. In 2007 two observational studies were published that demonstrated an impressive effect of spironolactone when added to a drug regimen that included an angiotensin-blocking agent, a CCB and a diuretic. The use of spironolactone is likely to increase as a result of these findings.

The main problem with spironolactone is its side effects. Most of them can be kept to a minimum if only low doses are used. In men spironolactone can cause breast tenderness and even breast enlargement. This almost precludes the use of this drug in men. Spironolactone has no effects on women's breasts.

The other problem is related to the mechanism of action of spironolactone. It causes potassium retention. In low doses the rise in serum potassium is small and of no great significance. Larger rises in serum potassium are seen when this agent is used in combination with an angiotensin-blocking agent such as lisinopril or losartan. Occasionally the serum potassium rises to above 6.0 millimoles per litre and could cause serious problems with heart rhythm. This is mainly a problem in patients receiving these agents for heart failure rather than hypertension. It is also common in patients with impaired kidney function and those with diabetes. All people receiving spironolactone should have their kidney function and serum potassium checked regularly.

A more selective aldosterone receptor antagonist is now available. This is eplerenone. It has been shown to reduce mortality in patients with heart failure and, being a selective antagonist, it does not cause breast problems in men. There is almost no information on eplerenone in people with resistant hypertension.

Amiloride is a potassium-retaining diuretic that is chemically unrelated to spironolactone. Its only mode of action is to stimulate the kidneys to remove salt and water while retaining potassium. It is not very effective when used alone but is sometimes used together with a thiazide diuretic. There has recently been some interest in using amiloride as a fourth-line drug in resistant hypertension.

Other antihypertensive drugs

The three drug classes described above are the recommended first-, second- and third-line drugs for treating hypertension. There are several other types of blood pressure-lowering drugs that may be used in special circumstances:

- The beta-adrenergic receptor blockers (beta blockers)

- The alpha blockers

- Centrally acting drugs

- Direct vasodilators.

The beta blockers

The beta blockers were introduced in the 1960s for the treatment of angina (heart pain on exercise). They were later shown to improve survival in patients who have had a heart attack and those with heart failure. They remain important drugs in the treatment of heart disease.

Beta blockers

- Acebutolol
- Atenolol
- Bisoprolol
- Carvedilol
- Celiprolol
- Labetalol
- Metoprolol
- Nebivolol

They work by blocking the actions of noradrenaline and adrenaline, which prepare the body for emergency situations – the so-called 'fight or flight' response. These powerful hormones open some blood vessels and narrow others, controlling blood flow to vital organs such as the heart. They speed up the heart and make it pump more forcibly. The beta blockers stop all this happening, so they slow the heart, lessen the force of its contractions and lower the blood pressure.

How beta blockers work

Beta blockers block the binding of noradrenaline on to the adrenoreceptors on the heart, so slowing the heart, reducing the force of its contractions and therefore lowering blood pressure.

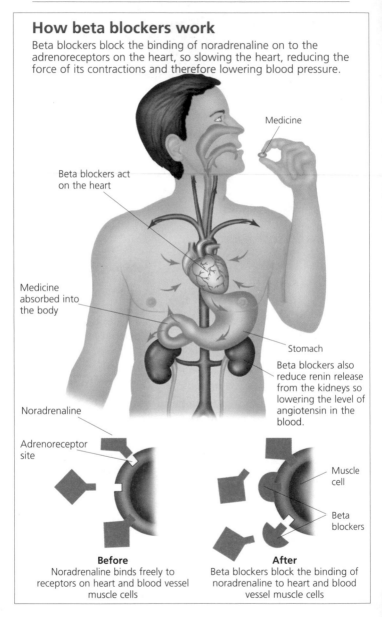

Medicine

Beta blockers act on the heart

Medicine absorbed into the body

Stomach

Beta blockers also reduce renin release from the kidneys so lowering the level of angiotensin in the blood.

Noradrenaline

Adrenoreceptor site

Muscle cell

Beta blockers

Before
Noradrenaline binds freely to receptors on heart and blood vessel muscle cells

After
Beta blockers block the binding of noradrenaline to heart and blood vessel muscle cells

These drugs also work by blocking the release of renin from the kidneys, thus reducing circulating levels of the hormone angiotensin II, which constricts blood vessels and raises blood pressure. This is probably the main mechanism of their antihypertensive effect. The beta blockers (particularly atenolol) became the most popular antihypertensive drugs worldwide. They were much more tolerable than the other drugs available at the time.

The main side effect was lethargy. Patients often did not notice this at first, so most were happy to continue to take them. They may also cause vivid dreams and reduced exercise capability. Again this was initially mild and not bothersome. These side effects became more obvious when patients stopped taking their beta blocker; many then reported that they now felt more energetic and slept better.

As the beta blockers work by reducing circulating levels of renin and angiotensin, it came as no surprise that they, similar to the angiotensin-blocking drugs described above, are less effective in older patients and people of African origin.

The beta blockers also work on the beta receptors in the airways. They can provoke asthma attacks in people who already have this condition.

When the newer blood pressure-lowering drugs (the angiotensin-blocking drugs and the calcium channel blockers) became available in the late 1990s, two major comparative studies were set up to investigate whether they were better, as good or not as good as the beta blockers at preventing heart attacks and strokes. The first, the Losartan Intervention For Endpoints (LIFE) trial, was published in 2002. In this trial 9,000 hypertensive patients were randomly allocated to receive either the

ARB, losartan, or the beta blocker, atenolol. Where necessary to control the blood pressure, the thiazide diuretic hydrochlorothiazide was added in. In this trial losartan was associated with 25 per cent fewer strokes and 25 per cent fewer cases of new-onset diabetes. It remains uncertain whether this is a beneficial effect of losartan or an adverse effect of atenolol.

In 2005, the Anglo Scandinavian Cardiac Outcome Trial (ASCOT) was published. This trial in 19,000 hypertensive patients compared a regimen based on atenolol (beta blocker) with a regimen based on amlodipine (calcium channel blocker). The patients on atenolol developed 23 per cent more strokes and 30 per cent more new-onset diabetes than the patients on amlodipine.

These two large comparative studies, together with an increasing awareness of the insidious side effects of the beta blockers substantially influenced the views of hypertension experts. In 2006 joint guidelines issued by the British Hypertension Society (BHS) and the National Institute for Health and Clinical Excellence (NICE) recommended that beta blockers should not be used as the first-, second- or third-line drugs for the treatment of hypertension, unless there is concurrent heart disease.

So the beta blockers are now back where they belong, as an important treatment for patients with established heart disease. They should not be used in hypertensive people with no heart disease (the majority).

If you are being treated with a beta blocker for raised blood pressure, you should not stop taking this drug without first discussing this with your doctor. In many people it may be sensible to phase out the beta blocker rather than stop abruptly. Also it will usually be necessary for your doctor to prescribe an alternative drug in one of the three classes described at the start of this section.

Alpha blockers
These work by blocking the action of the hormone, adrenaline, on muscles that make up the walls of small blood vessels. Adrenaline makes the blood vessels constrict and pushes up blood pressure. Blocking these receptors makes the blood vessels relax and blood pressure fall. As a result of this, they can also cause dizziness, especially when you stand up suddenly, but, other than that, they have few side effects.

Alpha blockers
● Doxazosin
● Indoramin
● Prazosin
● Terazosin

The early alpha blockers needed to be given three times a day and caused side effects of dizziness, light-headedness and a dry mouth. More recently two alpha blockers have been introduced that can be taken once daily: doxazosin and terazosin. They are safe but may still cause some dizziness in some individuals. Alpha-receptor blockers work on other parts of the body as well as the blood pressure. They have been shown, in particular, to relax the bladder and this is useful for elderly men with enlarged prostates who have difficulty in passing water. By contrast they can cause stress incontinence or loss of bladder control among women. This common but under-recognised side effect of alpha blockers almost precludes their use in women.

Alpha blockers have been shown to be associated with a slight improvement in sexual function in some men. For this reason alpha blockers may occasionally

How alpha blockers work

Alpha blockers block the binding of noradrenaline on to the alpha-adrenoreceptors in the muscles that make up the walls of blood vessels; this causes the vessels to dilate and therefore reduce blood pressure.

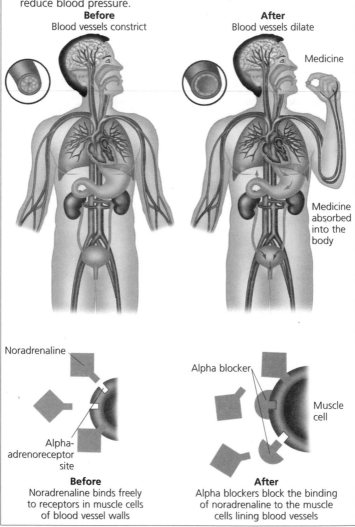

Before
Blood vessels constrict

After
Blood vessels dilate

Medicine

Medicine absorbed into the body

Noradrenaline

Alpha blocker

Muscle cell

Alpha-adrenoreceptor site

Before
Noradrenaline binds freely to receptors in muscle cells of blood vessel walls

After
Alpha blockers block the binding of noradrenaline to the muscle cells lining blood vessels

be used as a first-line therapy in men with erectile dysfunction who have difficulty in obtaining or maintaining an erection, as well as men with difficulties in passing urine due to a large prostate.

In the year 2000, a large American study showed that the thiazide-type diuretic chlortalidone was better than doxazosin (alpha blocker) at preventing heart failure. This trial remains a little controversial and some authorities do not accept these conclusions. However, the general body of opinion is that the alpha-blocking drugs should be used for patients with more severe resistant hypertension, in addition to other therapies.

Centrally acting drugs

The two drugs in this class are methyldopa and moxonidine. They work by acting on the part of the brain that controls blood pressure. Although they saved

Centrally acting drugs
• Clonidine
• Methyldopa
• Moxonidine

many lives in the past, this class of drugs is very rarely used now. Although it is entirely safe it does tend to cause tiredness, lethargy and even, when used in high dose, depression.

Newer drugs, which work in different ways, have fewer side effects and are equally safe, so methyldopa is now usually used only when other drugs have been found to be ineffective in reducing blood pressure.

Methyldopa is still prescribed for pregnant women for whom it is known to be safe. For very good reasons, doctors tend to prescribe drugs in pregnancy only if they have been available for a great many years. This is simply because the world experience is such that they can be confident that there will be no adverse effects on the developing baby. There is good evidence that methyldopa is safe in pregnancy. If you are given it while you're pregnant, however, you will probably change to another type of drug after the birth if your blood pressure still requires treatment.

More recently, a new centrally acting drug called moxonidine has been introduced. This appears to have fewer side effects than methyldopa, but there are no long-term outcome studies on its efficacy at preventing heart attacks or strokes. For this reason moxonidine tends to be used as an add-in fourth agent in patients whose blood pressures are uncontrolled with conventional medication. At the present stage of knowledge, moxonidine should not be used in pregnancy.

Direct vasodilators

These are hydralazine and minoxidil. They are rarely used nowadays. Hydralazine is occasionally used by injection or by mouth for severe hypertension in pregnancy. On a long-term basis it can cause a disease called lupus, which resembles rheumatoid arthritis. Minoxidil is a very powerful vasodilator that is effective in resistant hypertension. It causes ankle swelling and a fast pulse. With the advent of the newer drugs described earlier, it is hardly ever needed.

Combination therapies

As explained earlier, more than half the people with hypertension need to take more than one drug to control it, but usually this will mean taking a maximum of four tablets a day, sometimes fewer. Certain combinations of drugs are more effective than others.

Although there are many exceptions, in general the beta blockers and ACE inhibitors are best given with either thiazide diuretics or calcium channel blockers. There is often not much to be gained by combining a beta blocker with an ACE inhibitor or combining a thiazide diuretic with a calcium channel blocker.

If you are one of the minority of people who need three drugs to control your blood pressure, then there are probably no important drug interactions. It is considered best to use two or more blood pressure-lowering drugs in lower doses rather than any one drug in a high dose. All drugs can be taken together once daily so even quadruple therapy requires only four pills taken together. To help patients who require combination therapies, there are several blood pressure-lowering tablets that contain two different drugs that work well together (for example, Zestoretic and Cozaar-Comp).

British Hypertension Society guidelines

The British Hypertension Society (BHS) has published very sensible guidelines on the choice of drugs for patients with high blood pressure. These were updated in 2006 and again in 2011. In general younger patients, and those with diabetes, should be prescribed ACE inhibitors or ARBs as a first line, whereas older patients and African origin patients should be given calcium channel blockers (CCBs).

As 75 per cent of all hypertensive patients need more than one drug to control their blood pressure, the BHS guidelines also make sensible suggestions about what drug to add in. It is usual to add an ACE inhibitor or an ARB to a CCB and to add a CCB to an ACE inhibitor or an ARB. If the combination of an angiotensin blocker with a CCB is insufficient to bring the blood pressure to below 140/80 mmHg, the

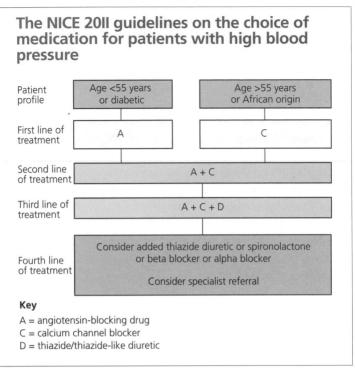

The NICE 2011 guidelines on the choice of medication for patients with high blood pressure

Patient profile	Age <55 years or diabetic	Age >55 years or African origin
First line of treatment	A	C
Second line of treatment	A + C	
Third line of treatment	A + C + D	
Fourth line of treatment	Consider added thiazide diuretic or spironolactone or beta blocker or alpha blocker Consider specialist referral	

Key

A = angiotensin-blocking drug
C = calcium channel blocker
D = thiazide/thiazide-like diuretic

guidelines suggest that the next step is to add in a thiazide diuretic. The scheme is illustrated in the figure above (using the 2011 guidelines from the National Institute for Health and Clinical Excellence [NICE]). In a nutshell it is A or C, A + C, A + C + D.

Thus beta blockers were removed from this recommendation and the thiazides were downgraded to be a third-line agent in 2011.

Hypertension resistant to triple therapy with A + C + D

There is no consensus on what to do if the blood pressure remains above 140/80 mmHg despite triple therapy in the top doses as described above. However, some suggestions are made here:

- Is your blood pressure truly resistant? It is possible that you have a white coat effect so that your pressure is only raised when you see your doctor. It is worthwhile doing 24-hour ambulatory monitoring (ABPM) or, failing that, home self-monitoring of your blood pressure. You may find that your pressure is fine the moment you leave your health centre.

- Are you sometimes forgetting to take your pills? Complicated tablet regimens are difficult to stick to. Your doctor may be able to simplify your drug regimen without loss of effectiveness. Sometimes it is possible to take two drugs in a single tablet.

- Are you adhering to a healthy diet? You should make big efforts to reduce your salt intake, take more exercise and where relevant moderate your alcohol intake.

- Are you overweight? If you lose 2 pounds in weight your pressure should fall by 1 mmHg. Lose 10 pounds and your pressure will fall by 5 mmHg.

- Are we missing an underlying medical cause for your hypertension? Your doctor may opt to refer you to a hypertension specialist to make sure that you do not have an underlying kidney or hormone disease causing your hypertension.

If you truly have resistant hypertension then it will be necessary to add in a fourth drug. There are several possibilities:

- Increase the dose of the thiazide diuretic (for example, bendroflumethiazide 5 mg)

- Add in the aldosterone antagonist, spironolactone, 25 mg

- Add in the alpha blocker, doxazosin 2 to 4 mg daily

- Add in a beta blocker (for example, bisoprolol 2.5 mg)

- Add in moxonidine 200 to 400 µg daily.

It will be clear from the several possibilities listed that there is insufficient information on which drug combination to give. The policy of this author is:

Men: A + C + D + doxazosin

Women: A + C + D + spironolactone

People of African–Caribbean and Asian origin
The African–Caribbean community

Hypertension is very common among people who are of African–Caribbean origin. In the USA, it is twice as common as in the white and Hispanic populations. The picture is much the same in the UK. By sharp contrast, in rural Africa hypertension is relatively uncommon but is very common in town and city dwellers. There is reasonably good evidence that the increased prevalence of hypertension in the African-origin community in the UK and the USA is related to salt intake. In Africa, with increasing urbanisation, there is a sharp increase in salt intake with a concurrent reduction in potassium intake (from fruit and vegetables), and both these effects are contributing to the rise in people's blood pressure.

Usually, with urbanisation, there is also a sharp increase in body weight, further aggravating a rise in blood pressure.

Within the UK and the USA, there is less convincing evidence that people of African–Caribbean origin consume more salt than anyone else, although in the USA they tend to have a diet that is low in potassium because they eat fewer pieces of fresh fruit and vegetables. It does appear, however, that people of African–Caribbean origin may be more sensitive to a given salt load than those from different racial backgrounds.

Possibly as a result of the increased sensitivity to salt, people of African–Caribbean origin who have hypertension have been shown to have lower levels of the hormones renin and angiotensin II in their blood. This is important because, as we have seen, some of the drugs that lower blood pressure do so by blocking the effects of these particular hormones. It will come as no surprise therefore that these drugs are less effective in people who have low renin and angiotensin levels in the first place. So, although ACE inhibitors and probably the angiotensin receptor blockers (ARBs) may not work as well for you if you are of African–Caribbean origin, drugs that work in a different way, such as thiazide diuretics, calcium channel blockers, alpha blockers and possibly the centrally acting drugs, offer effective alternatives.

Another important factor is that diabetes is three times more common in African–Caribbean people in the UK compared with white people, and diabetes and hypertension commonly occur together. If you have both, your risk of developing cardiovascular disease is higher. This means that your doctor is likely to want you to start on antihypertensive drugs, even though your blood pressure may be only very slightly raised. In fact, the current view is that everyone, from whatever ethnic background, who has both diabetes and hypertension, should receive this type of treatment if their blood pressure consistently exceeds 140/80 mmHg.

In the UK, and to a lesser extent in the USA, coronary heart disease (that is, heart attacks and angina) is relatively less common in people of African–Caribbean origin. On the other hand, strokes and kidney failure are more common. The reasons for these ethnic differences are not entirely certain, but, from a practical point of view, if you do belong to the African–Caribbean community, you need to take on board the importance of:

- restricting your salt intake

- having your blood pressure measured regularly

- being prepared to start (and keep taking) drug treatment if your blood pressure is consistently high.

There is good news, however. There is evidence that African–Caribbean patients with hypertension derive more benefit from a low-salt diet than patients of European origin.

Despite the fact that the ACE inhibitors and ARBs are less effective in patients of African origin there is evidence that these drugs are effective at preventing kidney damage in African–Caribbean patients who have pre-existing kidney disease. This is thought to result from a direct action of these drugs on the kidney and is probably not related to the effects on blood pressure. These patients often also need a thiazide diuretic or a calcium channel blocker in order to control their blood pressure.

The Asian community

People of south Asian origin who live in this country are more prone to develop hypertension than their white neighbours. This is thought to be related to a greater tendency to be overweight and to a higher frequency of developing diabetes. The rates of coronary heart disease (angina and heart attacks) in Asian communities in the UK are very high, possibly in part because some individuals consume large amounts of fatty foods.

As with the African–Caribbean community, however, the ethnic difference remains partly unexplained. People from an Asian background do not seem, on the basis of current evidence, to respond any differently from white people to the various classes of antihypertensive drugs.

Other ethnic groups

At present we know relatively little about hypertension and the risks associated with it as regards other ethnic groups in the UK. Some people of Chinese origin consume large amounts of salt in their food and this may explain the high incidence of strokes in both China and Japan. There is almost no information on this topic from the UK. Having said that, the advice given earlier about cutting down salt is worth following, whatever your ethnic background. There is no evidence that any of the Oriental or Asian herbs or spices are harmful in any way. Be careful, however, about Oriental herbal remedies that are imported from China. Some are very toxic and there is no quality control of their contents.

Aspirin

Low-dose aspirin (75 mg once daily) has been seen to improve survival in patients who have had a heart attack or a stroke. There is good evidence that it is also useful in people who are at very high cardiovascular risk. The role of aspirin in people with high blood pressure but no other risk factors remains uncertain. Only one dedicated aspirin trial in 19,000 patients, half of whom received aspirin and half received dummy tablets, showed no benefits in the reduction of stroke. There were 45 fewer coronary complications but this rather unimpressive reduction was offset by the development of 52 more stomach haemorrhages.

The general view is that all hypertensive patients who have heart disease or a history of a stroke should take aspirin, but only if their blood pressures are well controlled. Similarly hypertensive patients who are at high cardiovascular risk, by virtue of high cholesterol levels or cigarette smoking, should take aspirin.

In the remainder of people with hypertension, but no other risk factors, the benefits of aspirin are small and there is an increased chance of developing a gastric haemorrhage.

Cholesterol-lowering drugs

The most commonly used cholesterol-lowering drugs are the statins (for example, simvastatin and atorvastatin). They have been shown to increase survival in heart attack patients and people with no heart disease but who are at high risk. This will include almost all people with high blood pressure, even if their blood cholesterol levels are not raised. This last comment needs to be explained.

In the Anglo-Scandinavian Cardiac Outcomes Trial (ASCOT), there were 10,000 patients with hypertension, who were at high risk of a stroke or heart attack, but whose blood cholesterol levels were not raised (below 6.5 mmol/litre). Half were given a statin and half received dummy tablets. This trial had to be discontinued after about three years: the patients receiving the statin had a highly significant reduction of both stroke and coronary complications.

So we now know that a very large proportion of people with raised blood pressure should be taking a statin. The only exceptions are those whose total cardiovascular risk is below 20 per cent in the next 10 years (see the colour charts on pages 150–2). These are mainly people with hypertension and no other risk factors who are less than 50 years of age. And that is a minority.

The universal benefits of a healthy lifestyle

The lifestyle advice is the same for everyone: a high-fat, high-salt, low fruit and vegetable diet is bad for your cardiovascular health whereas a low-fat, low-salt, high fruit and vegetable diet is beneficial and will help to protect you against ill health in general and cardiovascular disease in particular. Whatever ethnic group you belong to, you should also avoid drinking excessive amounts of alcohol and make a point of taking more exercise.

KEY POINTS

- There is a wide choice of antihypertensive drugs

- All antihypertensive drugs are roughly equally effective

- About half of all people who are hypertensive need two or more drugs to control their blood pressure

- The more modern drugs have fewer side effects

Special cases

Pregnant women

Your blood pressure usually stays the same or falls a little while you are pregnant. Some women actually find out that it is high during pregnancy but this is because it has been that way for some time, and they haven't had it checked before. In this situation, it's purely coincidental and not really related to pregnancy; it just happens to be detected while you are pregnant. Its management is the same as for anyone else who is diagnosed with hypertension, although the choice of drugs may be different.

About 25 per cent of women expecting their first baby develop slightly raised blood pressure in the last third of pregnancy. If they do not have any kidney damage and no protein appears in the urine on testing, then drug therapy may not be given to bring the pressure down. The significance of mildly raised blood pressure in pregnancy is uncertain, but careful monitoring is crucial.

Pre-eclampsia

Hypertension that develops in the second half of pregnancy, but with no protein appearing in the urine, is sometimes referred to as gestational hypertension. It is now becoming apparent that gestational hypertension may really be just a very mild form of pre-eclampsia.

Pre-eclampsia is potentially very serious for you and your baby. It affects about five per cent of women in the second half of their first pregnancies, and is defined as a blood pressure of over 160/90; a urine test will usually show that you have protein in your urine. If undetected it can progress into a very serious condition called eclampsia, in which the woman has fits and both mother and baby are in danger. Hospital admission and specialised treatment are necessary. The cause of this condition is not yet fully understood or preventable. Pre-eclampsia is less common in second and third pregnancies (if the pregnancy is by the same father).

This is the reason why your blood pressure and urine are checked every time you attend the antenatal clinic. If you have been prescribed antihypertensive drug treatment for the first time while you are pregnant, you will probably be able to come off it once your baby is about two weeks old, but your doctors will want you to come back for regular check-ups. Many women who have had hypertension in their first pregnancy will have no further trouble next time round.

Blood pressure treatment in pregnancy

In pregnancy, there is a severe limit to the choice of blood pressure-lowering drugs. Methyldopa (centrally acting) is known to be entirely safe and labetalol may be safe. Atenolol (beta blocker) has been shown in three studies to be associated with reduced growth of the baby and is no longer recommended in women who are pregnant or women who are likely to become pregnant.

The ACE inhibitors and the angiotensin receptor blockers should never be used in pregnancy under any circumstances. They should also never be used in women who are preparing to have children. There are reports that ACE inhibitors may cause birth defects although a recent large study from England could not confirm this risk

If the pressure is resistant to therapy, then nifedipine (calcium channel blocker) may be added in, although there is only limited information about its use.

Women who have had raised blood pressure in pregnancy, which has settled once the baby has been delivered, are now known to have a greater chance of developing hypertension and its complications in later life. For this reason, any woman who has had hypertension in pregnancy should be seen once a year by the family doctor or practice nurse.

People with chest diseases

The most important point is that you can't take beta-blocker drugs if you have any form of wheeze, asthma or similar breathing difficulties, but there is no problem as regards other antihypertensive drugs. The ACE inhibitors can cause a dry, irritating cough, but this is not usually associated with breathlessness. The cough will disappear once you stop taking the tablets and there are plenty of alternative treatments.

People with angina

If you have this condition, you will need detailed

assessment, including measurement of your serum cholesterol levels and, if necessary, cholesterol-lowering drugs. Beta-blocker drugs may be particularly helpful in reducing the frequency of angina attacks, but you will need to be carefully monitored by your doctor while taking them. Most patients with angina should be referred to a hospital-based heart specialist for consideration of detailed X-rays of the heart (coronary angiography).

After a heart attack

After a heart attack you may benefit from taking lipid-lowering drugs such as simvastatin to lower your cholesterol levels so as to minimise the risk of further heart attacks. ACE inhibitors and beta blockers may have additional advantages from your point of view because, as well as controlling your blood pressure, they make the heart work less hard and help to protect the heart muscle from further damage. Your doctor will usually recommend that you take low-dose aspirin every day.

After a stroke

If you have had the misfortune to have a stroke, lowering your blood pressure rapidly may be harmful but, on a longer-term basis, keeping your blood pressure under careful control does reduce the risk of a recurrence. The choice of drug treatment will be up to your doctor and the fact that you have had a stroke doesn't mean that you can't take some types or that others would be especially appropriate. If tests show that your stroke was caused by a cerebral thrombosis (blood clot in the brain), as opposed to a cerebral haemorrhage, then you will usually be prescribed aspirin in a low dose.

Anxiety and depression

If you have a tendency to be depressed or worried about your hypertension, it is worth remembering that antihypertensive drug therapy has been the great medical success story of the last 50 years because it brings about an impressive reduction in heart attack and stroke.

Patients who tend to be over-anxious or who get panic attacks are sometimes given a low dose of a beta blocker. This treatment can reduce the severity of anxiety. Beta blockers do not, however, have any mood-altering effects; they are not officially psychiatric drugs and are in no way habit forming (unlike Valium/diazepam).

The older beta blockers, such as propranolol and the centrally acting drug methyldopa, may not be suitable for you because they can be associated with depression, lethargy and tiredness, so if you have a tendency towards depression these drugs are best avoided. The thiazide diuretics and the newer classes of antihypertensive drugs appear to have no effects on mood.

If your depression is being treated with lithium therapy, you should not take thiazide diuretics for hypertension because your blood lithium levels may then rise to potentially hazardous levels.

The contraceptive pill

Most oral contraceptive pills cause a tiny and unimportant rise in blood pressure. However, the diastolic blood pressure rises to more than 90 mmHg in about 5 per cent of women – usually those who are older, overweight and with a past history of slightly raised blood pressure readings. Only in rare circumstances can the contraceptive pill alone cause severe hypertension with a level that requires treatment.

There is evidence that the newer, low-dose, combined oral preparations and the progesterone-only pills cause a smaller rise in blood pressure than the older, high-dose, combined preparations. You may be able to take the combined oral contraceptive pill even if you have hypertension, provided that you are carefully monitored by your doctor or practice nurse. It is particularly important to avoid becoming overweight. Many of the complications that may result from taking oral contraceptive pills affect older women who are also cigarette smokers.

HRT

The amount of oestrogen in hormone replacement therapy (HRT) is much smaller than that in the oral contraceptive pill. In the past doctors have been somewhat cautious about prescribing HRT for women with hypertension, but recent surveys suggest that this is quite safe provided that you are carefully monitored by your doctor. Hypertension on its own is not a reason not to take HRT, but you do have to avoid putting on a lot of weight, which can sometimes happen with this treatment. There is no evidence that HRT in any way interferes with antihypertensive drugs.

Early surveys suggested that HRT might be associated with a reduced risk of heart attack and stroke. Unfortunately well-conducted placebo-controlled (dummy) drug trials have shown that this is not the case. In fact there was a very small excess of heart disease and stroke in women taking HRT. As a result of these findings most clinicians feel that

HRT should not be given in an attempt to prevent heart disease, but should be given only to prevent the unpleasant symptoms associated with the menopause (change of life). We would no longer recommend HRT to be given for more than about five years, unless it is really necessary to relieve unpleasant symptoms.

Children

Severely raised blood pressures in children are rare and are usually associated with significant kidney conditions; such children should be seen in specialist children's hospitals. Overweight children and those with a strong family history of hypertension may have slightly raised blood pressure. If you yourself have hypertension, you should be aware that your children are at risk of developing it too. Try to ensure that their diet is as low in salt as possible and, in particular, don't let them eat too many crisps or other salted snacks or convenience foods such as burgers. It's also important not to let them get fat.

Very rarely, high blood pressure can be the result of autosomal dominant polycystic kidney disease. This is usually diagnosed in adult life but a parent with the condition needs to know that there is a chance that 50 per cent of his or her children are likely to have this condition. If you have autosomal dominant polycystic kidney disease you should arrange for your children to be screened for this condition.

Diabetes mellitus

Since 1995, there have been some major advances in our understanding of the treatment of patients with diabetes. More than half of all people with diabetes have raised blood pressure and the value of controlling blood pressure is impressive. People with diabetes are prone to two sorts of vascular damage:

- microvascular (small vessel) damage to the kidneys, eyes and nerves

- macrovascular (large vessel) damage to the arteries of the legs, brain and heart.

As a result of this and other findings, the British Hypertension Society now recommends that people with diabetes should have their blood pressure reduced, if possible, to below 130/80 mmHg.

Two types of diabetes

It's worth remembering that there are also two types of diabetes, with very little overlap. There is type 1 (insulin-dependent) diabetes, which starts in childhood or early life. Patients with this form of diabetes are prone to develop microvascular damage to the kidneys and retina. Almost all such patients are treated with insulin injections. Once the kidneys become involved, the blood pressure usually rises and antihypertensive treatment is necessary.

By contrast, type 2 (non-insulin-dependent) diabetes commonly occurs in older people who are often overweight and already have hypertension. These people are more prone to heart attacks and strokes as a result of macrovascular damage. Treatment may be initially with diet alone or oral antidiabetic tablets, and a minority of patients are also given insulin injections. In both forms of diabetes, the angiotensin-converting enzyme (ACE) inhibitors and the angiotensin receptor blockers have been shown to prevent or delay renal damage even if the blood pressure is not raised.

There is now good evidence that both blood pressure reduction and the lowering of blood cholesterol levels in people with diabetes do lead to the prevention of heart attacks and strokes. A very important British study published in 1998 showed that lowering of blood pressure to below 140/85 mmHg in type 2 diabetes was extremely beneficial.

All people with diabetes therefore need to have their cholesterol checked and reduced if it is raised. In addition, it is necessary to try to control blood sugar as well as possible with either tablets or insulin.

Furthermore, it is crucially important to bring down the blood pressure. There is good evidence that a low-salt diet is particularly beneficial in patients with type 2 diabetes and this diet also enhances the effect of some blood pressure-lowering drugs.

To achieve good blood pressure control in patients with diabetes, it is almost invariably necessary to give at least two, and sometimes three, different antihypertensive drugs. Most specialists in diabetes now prefer to use ACE inhibitors or the angiotensin receptor blockers as first-line drugs because they have been shown to delay diabetic kidney damage.

In 2007 a major international trial of the use of blood pressure-lowering drugs in diabetes (the ADVANCE trial) was published. This showed that the treatment of patients with diabetes with a combination of the ACE inhibitor drug, perindopril, and the thiazide-like diuretic, indapamide, was associated with a reduction of the vascular complications of diabetes. This benefit was seen both in patients with hypertension and in those with normal blood pressures. This trial has confirmed many in their view that practically all people with diabetes should be receiving an ACE inhibitor or, if this is not tolerated, an angiotensin receptor blocker (ARB).

It is then usual to add in a calcium channel blocker if necessary. The thiazide diuretics at high doses can worsen diabetes; this tended to make them less popular in the past. However, we now know that, used in the correct dose, these diuretics are beneficial in patients with diabetes, usually when they are used as add-in therapy.

There is increasing consensus that, in type 2 diabetes, the top priorities are to treat the blood pressure and the cholesterol. Lowering blood sugar has some benefits also, but blood pressure and cholesterol are more important.

Elderly people

Some years ago, elderly people were seen as a separate subgroup who needed to be treated differently from younger people, but this view is now known to be spurious. As you get older your blood pressures rises and the risk of heart attack and strokes becomes correspondingly greater. Recent treatment trials have shown that antihypertensive treatment is particularly effective in older people and a great many heart attacks and strokes can be prevented. Older people do have a higher frequency of other conditions, including diabetes and arthritis, and, if you have a condition such as these, you may require different antihypertensive drugs.

Otherwise, treatment for hypertension is the same, whatever your age. If your blood pressure is persistently greater than 160/100 mmHg even after you have followed the advice on lifestyle changes, you will need to start taking antihypertensive drugs.

There is a trend for the thiazide diuretics and the calcium channel blockers to be more effective and the ACE inhibitors and the beta blockers less effective in older patients. Sometimes you may need to take two different drugs in low dose rather than any one drug in high dose.

You can be reassured that controlling your blood pressure with drugs is particularly effective at preventing strokes. There's no reason why you shouldn't lead a normal, active life while making sure that you follow a healthy diet which does not contain too much salt, but contains adequate amounts of potassium-rich fruit and vegetables. The benefits of treating hypertension in elderly people are impressive at all ages.

As reported on page 87, 2008 saw the publication of a major treatment trial that was conducted in men and women aged over 80 years (HYVET). Until then there had been some uncertainty as to whether antihypertensive drug therapy was worthwhile in people of this age. The limited information available suggested that, although there seemed to be a reduction in strokes, this appeared to be offset by a slight increase in deaths from all causes. Clearly a dedicated trial to clarify this point was necessary. In HYVET, 3,845 people with hypertension were randomly allocated to receive either the thiazide-like diuretic, indapamide, together with the ACE inhibitor, perindopril, or matching dummy (placebo) tablets. The results were very impressive. Active treatment reduced strokes by 30 per cent and heart failure by 64 per cent, and there was a 21 per cent reduction in deaths from all causes. Drug side effects and adverse reactions were more common in the patients who were randomised to receive the dummy tablets.

This historic UK-based trial is almost certainly the last in which patients would be randomly allocated to receive active versus inactive treatment. Further trials of this design would now be considered ethically unjustifiable. We now know that all patients at all ages with hypertension need tablets to reduce their blood pressures.

KEY POINTS

■ Pregnant women need careful blood pressure assessment, and drug treatment is occasionally necessary

■ Concomitant heart disease, chest disease and diabetes influence choice of blood pressure-lowering drugs

■ Blood pressure in people aged over 65 is managed in exactly the same way as in younger people, and this definitely prevents heart attacks and strokes

Advances in hypertension research

The pace of medical research

The topic of blood pressure in general, and of hypertension in particular, has been the focus of a great deal of medical research since World War II. We are well served by huge population studies that have told us a lot about who is at risk of developing a heart attack or a stroke. They have drawn attention to the fact that hypertension is the most common chronic medical condition on this planet.

Blood pressure: a public health issue

The finding that people whose blood pressures are exactly average for their age are still at higher risk than those whose pressures are below average means that, if we are to do anything to reduce the numbers of people who develop heart, brain or kidney damage, we should do all we can to bring about a fall in the average blood pressure of the whole population. Thus blood pressure is a public health issue that can be solved by public health manoeuvres.

There is strong evidence that the average blood pressure of the population can be reduced by public health means. If the population average salt intake could be reduced, blood pressures would fall. The good news is that, in the UK there has been a reduction in average salt intake from ten grams to eight grams daily over the last decade. The target is to reduce salt intake down to six grams daily by 2015, and it is to be hoped that this will be achieved. Major food manufacturers and supermarkets are now cooperating but there is a lot to be done. Of interest, the World Health Organization (WHO) has recently suggested a target salt intake of five grams daily.

A frequent question asked is 'How much salt do we actually need?'. The answer is 'probably about two grams daily, on the basis of studies of chimpanzees and other primates in the wild and in captivity'. Humans are the only animals that add crystals of sodium chloride to their food.

Similarly, if we can manage to achieve a reversal of the rising tide of obesity, the whole population would benefit. Likewise, with rising alcohol consumption and with physical inactivity – both need reversing. As described earlier, the Dietary Approaches to Stop Hypertension (DASH) trial shows that dietary and lifestyle manoeuvres can reduce blood pressure in the short term, at least in people without hypertension as well as in those with hypertension. We need bigger and longer studies similar to DASH to investigate this issue further.

There is every reason to expect that the average blood pressures of populations in the developing world will rise with increasing urbanisation and the adoption of western-style, high-fat, high-salt diets, and a declining intake of vegetable products. Hypertension is becoming an increasing problem in Africa and Asia. The public health authorities in these developing countries need to avoid making the mistakes that we have made in the west.

On a public health basis, it is extremely unlikely that any new unexpected environmental or lifestyle factor will be discovered as a cause of the average blood pressure of the population, and the corresponding incidence of hypertension. In the INTERMAP population study, conducted in the UK, the USA, China and Japan, it was found that practically all of the differences of blood pressure within populations, and when comparing them, could be explained by variations of dietary and lifestyle factors. We know why blood pressures of populations rise and might one day hopefully fall.

Hypertension: a clinical condition

Turning to hypertension at a clinical level, we are also well served by the very large number of well-conducted trials of the treatment of hypertension, demonstrating significant reductions in heart attacks and strokes. The Hypertension in the Very Elderly Trial (HYVET) is almost certainly the last trial to compare the results of treatment versus no treatment. Up until about 2008 there was some anxiety that reducing blood pressure in very senior citizens might do more harm than good, with side effects of light-headedness and falls. The HYVET study showed the reverse: lowering blood pressure reduced strokes, heart failure and death rates. There is even some evidence that blood pressure lowering reduces or delays dementia, although the evidence on this is not yet watertight.

We know which patients benefit from blood pressure reduction and which do not. Perhaps the only groups for whom we need more information are children and young adults. It is unlikely that a long-term trial will ever be conducted here. The five- to ten-year risk is so small that the studies would need to recruit tens of thousands of patients to be given antihypertensive drugs or placebo for ten or more years, so the cost would be prohibitive.

Pre-hypertension

There have been two trials of the short-term drug treatment of pre-hypertension. Pre-hypertension is a condition in which a fit individual has a blood pressure in the upper part of the normal range. Such people do have about a 50 per cent chance of developing sustained hypertension within the next 5 to 10 years, so on a much longer-term basis they have a greater chance of developing heart disease and strokes. The logic of giving blood pressure-lowering drugs to people with pre-hypertension is undeniable, but the practicalities of the funding and management of a long-term trial seem insuperable. Also one must question whether labelling someone as having pre-hypertension, with the associated anxiety and inconvenience, might be counterproductive.

Hypertension and kidney disease

The observation that people with mildly impaired kidney function have a great deal more heart disease than one might expect, on the basis of the known cardiovascular risk factors, leads one to speculate whether there are as yet unknown mechanisms for such cardiovascular damage. More research into the mechanisms of vascular damage in kidney patients is needed.

Central blood pressure

There is increasing interest in the role of central blood pressure. The blood pressure that we measure in the clinic is in the upper arm and this differs from the central blood pressure, nearer to the heart, brain and kidneys. It seems that the central pressure is the one that really matters. Its measurement in routine clinical practice will soon be feasible and a great deal of research is going on in this field. Maybe one day it will be the central blood pressure that we will measure and treat.

Is there a need for newer antihypertensive drugs?

One must question whether we need more new types of blood pressure-lowering drugs. We now have an excellent choice of drugs that lower blood pressure while causing minimal side effects. Do we need more? The answer in the view of this author is 'probably not'. In general we know how to control blood pressure using the A + C + D regimen covered in earlier sections of this booklet. Would a newer class of antihypertensive drugs have any advantage over what we have already? Pharmacological innovation should be encouraged but at times of world financial recession should the priorities be elsewhere?

There is one field where we do need more information on how to treat the minority of patients who genuinely have blood pressures that cannot be controlled despite the A + C + D regimen. What is the best way to manage these patients? There is a need for a trial to help us know what drugs to add in as fourth-line agents. Maybe it will be a totally new agent not yet available or even developed.

Renal denervation: an exciting new advance

One very interesting area is the use of renal denervation to reduce blood pressure. In the 1950s, when blood pressure-lowering drugs were not available or intolerable to take, some patients were subjected to a thoracolumbar sympathectomy. This was a major surgical operation to cut out the sympathetic ganglia each side of the spinal columns. It did reduce blood pressure but was not feasible on a mass basis. With the advent of effective and tolerable blood pressure-lowering drugs, thoracolumbar sympathectomy was no longer needed.

Recently, there has been a rise in interest in blocking the sympathetic nerves supplying the kidneys. This can now be achieved without surgery by inserting a fine tube into the femoral artery in the groin and advancing it to enter the arteries supplying the kidneys. Once in place a pulse of high intensity ultrasound is discharged in the renal artery to ablate (destroy) the renal nerves on the outside of the artery. This can be performed with only the minimum of discomfort, usually without hospital admission. Preliminary research has demonstrated impressive and persisting reductions in blood pressure.

The role of renal denervation in the management of resistant hypertension will be the focus of much research in the next 10 years. However, one thing has become clear – many patients referred to specialist research centres for consideration of renal denervation treatment do not need it. In many, 24-hour blood pressure monitoring has shown that the blood pressure of many patients is under excellent control at all times except when they are visiting their doctor. This confirms the crucial importance of home blood pressure monitoring in the management of hypertension. Every patient should buy his or her own monitor, at a cost of under £20. One thing though – don't buy a wrist monitor, as they are not accurate.

Delivering good hypertension care: the next priority

There is a view that the golden age of hypertension research is drawing to a close. We know why people get raised blood pressures, we know whom to treat for raised blood pressure and we know how to treat it. The big question now is how to prevent hypertension in the first place, how to detect it when it does occur and how to deliver our effective treatments to the hundreds of millions of people worldwide. Now, that is a challenge.

Questions and answers

What is hypertension?
Hypertension is simply the state of having a blood pressure that is rather higher than average. If sustained, it can increase the risk of having a heart attack or a stroke.

Can anything be done about it?
Yes, lowering blood pressure definitely prevents heart attacks and strokes.

How can I find out whether I have hypertension?
The only way to find out whether you have high blood pressure is to have it measured by your doctor or practice nurse. I am afraid that there is no association between high blood pressure and any specific symptoms, including headache. All British adults should have a routine blood pressure check.

How can I get my blood pressure down?

You can help this by adopting a low-salt diet with plenty of fresh fruit and vegetables. In addition, you should try to avoid being overweight and consume only moderate amounts of alcohol.

What happens if this is not effective?

If your blood pressure cannot be lowered by non-drug therapies alone, then drug therapy is quite often necessary. There is, however, a wide choice of blood pressure-lowering drugs and it can almost be guaranteed that you will have no side effects.

The most important thing to remember is that, if your blood pressure is controlled, your risk of having a heart attack or stroke is greatly reduced.

Will I be able to stop my treatment?

You should discontinue antihypertensive drugs only under medical supervision with careful follow-up. Almost all patients need to take their drugs indefinitely for the rest of their lives. Even if you are able to stop the therapy, you will still have to be seen at least every few months for rechecking.

What is the cause of high blood pressure?

High blood pressure appears to result from the interplay of genetic (inherited) factors and lifestyle factors. There is a tendency in all western societies to consume large quantities of salt in food. In addition, being overweight and obesity can cause high blood pressure, as can excess alcohol consumption.

However, at the end of the day we do not know all the answers to this question. It is worth remembering that, in a very small minority of people, we can find underlying kidney diseases that are the cause of high blood pressure.

Should the blood pressure or its treatment affect my quality of life?

Definitely not. Modern drugs are virtually free of side effects. You are encouraged to return to a normal, active, busy and interesting life. Only people with very high blood pressure need to stop work, and even then only briefly.

How common is hypertension?

About ten million British citizens have raised blood pressure. Not all of them need drug treatment, but they all need careful supervision by their GP or practice nurse.

British Hypertension Society Cardiovascular Risk Prediction Charts

We are now able to calculate an individual person's risk of developing future coronary heart disease or stroke. In March 2004 the British Hypertension Society (BHS) published its fourth working party report on guidelines for managing hypertension. This appeared in the *Journal of Human Hypertension* with a shortened version in the *British Medical Journal*. With BHS IV there are colour charts where you can calculate your chances of developing heart attack or stroke in the next 10 years. Previous colour charts allowed only an estimation of the risk of heart attack and not stroke, so they were of limited value in managing people with hypertension who are also at risk of stroke. These predictions are based on a 54-year follow-up study in Framingham,

Massachusetts, USA. The Framingham prediction has been shown to translate fairly well into non-American populations. To calculate your cardiovascular disease (CVD) risk in the next 10 years, you will have to know your current systolic blood pressure (the higher value when blood is pumped out of the heart) and your serum total cholesterol divided by your high-density-lipoprotein (HDL)-cholesterol, which is often referred to as 'good cholesterol' (see page 149 for explanation). Then choose the right box of the colour charts on pages 150–2 according to your sex and age.

You can then see whether your CVD risk is high (more than 20 per cent over the next 10 years), moderate (10–20 per cent) or mild (less than 10 per cent). People who are at high risk may well need cholesterol-lowering drugs and the threshold for starting blood pressure treatment with drugs is 140/90 mmHg. With successful lowering of blood pressure and blood cholesterol the risk of CVD can be greatly reduced. These charts also demonstrate the enormous benefits for stopping smoking. The main problems with these charts is that they are not helpful in patients who are at very high risk indeed of having either a heart attack or stroke. Also they do not take into account concurrent diabetes or the impact of a bad family history of cardiovascular disease. The other problem is it is uncertain how accurate they are in African–Caribbean and south Asian patients. However, they do provide a useful guide and draw attention to the importance of looking at all risk factors and not just the blood pressure.

Cholesterol

The cholesterol in our bodies comes from two sources: the diet and some that we make ourselves. To reach the body tissues, cholesterol must be carried in blood plasma in particles called 'lipoproteins'. Lipoproteins are a family of particles in which there are five main classes, all of which have slightly different functions. They get their names from their relative density; the two classes that are most important for cholesterol transport are low-density lipoprotein (LDL) and high-density lipoprotein (HDL). Most of the cholesterol in blood is in LDL particles, although the number of HDL particles is greater than the number of LDL ones. The reason for this is that HDL contains relatively more protein and less cholesterol in each particle.

Increasingly high blood levels of HDL are associated with lower risks of developing CHD, hence the view that HDL contains good cholesterol. The reasons for this are not absolutely clear, but possibly relate to the fact that HDL removes cholesterol from cells and carries it to the liver. Thus, HDL could prevent cholesterol accumulating in key sites such as arterial walls, lessening the risk of atherosclerosis. A further possibility for the protective effects of HDL is that it has antioxidant activity. Oxidation of LDL is thought to occur before the particles are taken up in arterial walls and there is some, although not convincing, evidence that antioxidants may prevent this change occurring in LDL particles, and therefore protect against the development of atherosclerosis.

Calculation of cardiovascular disease (CVD) risk

To estimate an individual's absolute 10-year risk of developing CVD, find the table (see pages 151 and 152) for gender, smoking status (smoker/non-smoker) and age.

Then you need to know the person's:
Blood pressure
Total cholesterol (TC)
High-density lipoprotein (HDL) – if unknown assume 1.0 mmol/litre

For example, if you are a 50-year-old man, a non-smoker without diabetes and your:
- Blood pressure = 120/80 mmHg
- Total cholesterol (TC) = 6.2 mmol/litre
- HDL = 1.3 mmol/litre

Then:
Systolic blood pressure (SBP) = 120 mmHg
TC/HDL = 6.2/1.3 = 4.8

From the correct table (see pages 151–2) find the SBP on the vertical axis and the TC/HDL on the horizontal axis and read off the risk value (see example below).

In this case the risk of having a non-fatal or fatal heart attack or stroke is less than 10 per cent over the next 10 years.

Non-diabetic men

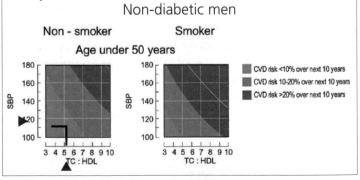

Cardiovascular Risk Prediction Charts

NON-DIABETIC MEN

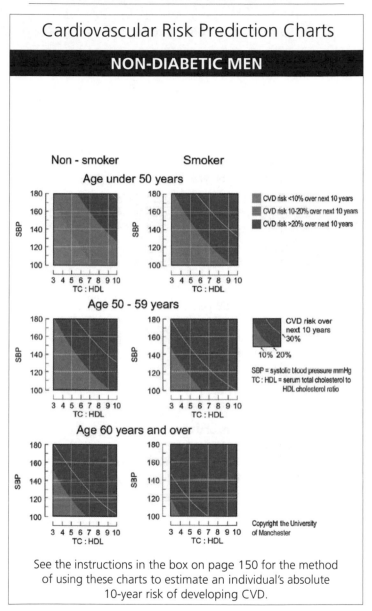

Non - smoker   **Smoker**

Age under 50 years

CVD risk <10% over next 10 years
CVD risk 10-20% over next 10 years
CVD risk >20% over next 10 years

Age 50 - 59 years

CVD risk over next 10 years
>30%
10% 20%

SBP = systolic blood pressure mmHg
TC : HDL = serum total cholesterol to HDL cholesterol ratio

Age 60 years and over

Copyright the University of Manchester

See the instructions in the box on page 150 for the method of using these charts to estimate an individual's absolute 10-year risk of developing CVD.

Cardiovascular Risk Prediction Charts

NON-DIABETIC WOMEN

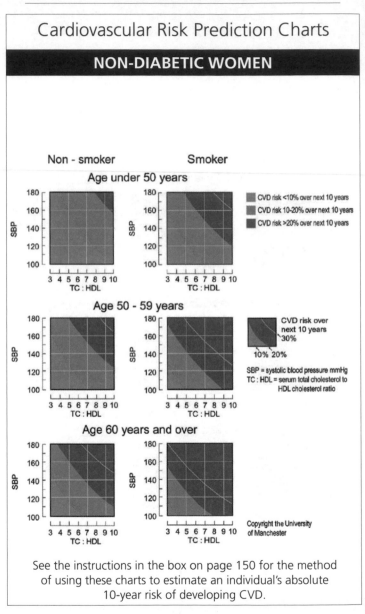

Non - smoker **Smoker**

Age under 50 years

- CVD risk <10% over next 10 years
- CVD risk 10-20% over next 10 years
- CVD risk >20% over next 10 years

Age 50 - 59 years

CVD risk over next 10 years
30%
10% 20%

SBP = systolic blood pressure mmHg
TC : HDL = serum total cholesterol to HDL cholesterol ratio

Age 60 years and over

Copyright the University of Manchester

See the instructions in the box on page 150 for the method of using these charts to estimate an individual's absolute 10-year risk of developing CVD.

Useful addresses

We have included the following organisations because, on preliminary investigation, they may be of use to the reader. However, we do not have first-hand experience of each organisation and so cannot guarantee the organisation's integrity. The reader must therefore exercise his or her own discretion and judgement when making further enquiries.

Benefit Enquiry Line
Tel: 0800 882200 (Mon–Fri 8am–6pm)
Textphone: 0800 243355
Website: www.gov.uk/benefit-enquiry-line

Government agency giving information and advice on sickness and disability benefits for people with disabilities and their carers.

Blood Pressure Association
Wolfson Institute, Charterhouse Square
London EC1M 6BQ
Tel: 020 7882 6255/5793

Information line: 0845 241 0989 (Mon–Fri 9am–midday)
Website: www.blood pressureuk.org

For the best internet advice. Regularly issues press statements when any new information becomes available and has advice leaflets on all aspects of hypertension (for example, pregnancy, renal disease, heart disease). Raises public awareness about, and offers information and support to, people affected by high blood pressure and health-care professionals. Has a wide selection of literature and membership scheme. Please send large A4 SAE and two first-class stamps for information.

British Heart Foundation
Greater London House
180 Hampstead Road
London NW1 7AW
Tel: 020 7554 0000
Heart helpline: 0300 330 3311 (local rate number, available Mon–Fri 9am–5pm, a free service for those seeking information on heart health issues)
BHF publications order line: 0870 600 6566 or order online
Website: www.bhf.org.uk

Funds research, promotes education and raises money to buy equipment to treat heart disease. Information and support available for people with heart conditions. Via Heartstart UK arranges training in emergency life-saving techniques for lay people.

British Hypertension Society
Clinical Sciences Wing, Glenfield Hospital, Groby Road,

Leicester LE3 9QB
Tel: 0116 250 2605
Website: www.bhsoc.org

Provides information to doctors, nurses, and other health professionals who work in the field of hypertension and cardiovascular disease. Has no patient leaflets; however, maintains a list of blood pressure monitors that is available to the public on request. This list is also on the website.

Chest, Heart & Stroke Scotland

Head office: Rosebery House, 9 Haymarket Terrace
Edinburgh EH12 5EZ
Tel: 0131 225 6963
Advice line: 0845 077 6000
Website: www.chss.org.uk

Funds research, provides care and support throughout Scotland, and has an advice line for professional advice from a trained nurse. Booklets, factsheets, DVDs and videos available free to patients and carers.

Circulation Foundation

35–43 Lincoln's Inn Fields
London WC2A 3PE
Tel: 020 7304 4779
Web: www.circulationfoundation.org.uk

Publishes a number of patient information leaflets to help identify and treat vascular illness. It also funds research into the prevention and causes of vascular disease.

HEART UK – The Cholesterol Charity
7 North Road
Maidenhead, Berks SL6 1PE
Helpline: 0845 450 5988 (Mon–Fri 10am–3pm)
Website: www.heartuk.org.uk

Offers information, advice and support to people
with coronary heart disease and especially those at
high risk of familial hypercholesterolaemia. Members
receive bimonthly magazine. Merged with British
Hyperlipidaemia Association in June 2002.

High Blood Pressure Foundation
Department of Medical Sciences, Western General
Hospital
Edinburgh EH4 2XU
Tel: 0131 332 9211 (office hours)
Website: www.dialdoncaster.co.uk

A registered charity dedicated to improving the basic
understanding, assessment, treatment and public
awareness of high blood pressure and, in so doing,
helping promote the welfare of people with high blood
pressure. Operates 'Friends' and covenant schemes to
assist with funding.

National Institute for Health and Clinical Excellence (NICE)
1st Floor, 10 Spring Gardens
London SW1A 2BU
Tel: 0845 003 7784
Website: www.nice.org.uk

Provides national guidance on the promotion of good health and treatment of ill-health. Patient information leaflets are available for each piece of guidance issued.

NHS Direct
Tel: 0845 4647 or 111 (24 hours, 365 days a year)
Website: www.nhsdirect.nhs.uk

Offers confidential health-care advice, information and referral service. A good first port of call for any health advice. In the next few months this telephone number is being replaced by the number 111 and the service will be NHS 111. The number should be used if help is needed fast but not as an emergency.

NHS Smoking Helpline
Freephone: 0800 022 4332 (9am–8pm, Mon–Fri, 11am–5pm Sat, Sun)
Website: http://smokefree.nhs.uk

Have advice, help and encouragement on giving up smoking. Specialist advisers available to offer ongoing support to those who genuinely are trying to give up smoking. Can refer to local branches.

Patients' Association
PO Box 935
Harrow, Middlesex HA1 3YJ
Helpline: 0845 608 4455
Tel: 020 8423 9111
Website: www.patients-association.com

Provides advice on patients' rights, leaflets and a directory of self-help groups.

Quit (Smoking Quitlines)

20 Curtain Road
London EC2A 3NF
Helpline: 0800 002200 (Mon–Fri 9am–8pm, Sat, Sun 10am–4pm)
Tel: 020 7539 1700
Website: www.quit.org.uk

Offers individual advice on giving up smoking in English and Asian languages. Talks to schools on smoking and pregnancy and can refer to local support groups. Runs training courses for professionals.

Stroke Association

Stoke Association House, 240 City Road
London EC1V 2PR
Tel: 020 7566 0300
Helpline: 0303 303 3100 (Mon–Fri 9am–5pm)
Website: www.stroke.org.uk

Funds research and provides information, now specialising only in strokes. Has local support groups.

Weight Watchers

Millennium House, Ludlow Road
Maidenhead SL6 2SL
Tel: 0845 345 1500
Website: www.weightwatchers.co.uk

Runs informal, yet structured, weekly meetings across the UK for people wanting to lose weight and learn more about living a healthy lifestyle. Guidance also available free with online programme.

Useful websites
BBC
www.bbc.co.uk/health
A helpful website: easy to navigate and offers lots of useful advice and information. Also contains links to other related topics.

Healthtalkonline
www.healthtalkonline.org
Website of the DIPEx charity.

NHS choices
www.nhs.uk/conditions
Government's patient information portal.

Patient UK
www.patient.co.uk
Patient care website.

The internet as a further source of information
After reading this book, you may feel that you would like further information on the subject. The internet is of course an excellent place to look and there are many websites with useful information about medical disorders, related charities and support groups.

For those who do not have a computer at home some bars and cafes offer facilities for accessing the internet. These are listed in the Yellow Pages under 'Internet Bars and Cafes' and 'Internet Providers'. Your local library offers a similar facility and has staff to help you find the information that you need.

It should always be remembered, however, that the internet is unregulated and anyone is free to set up a website and add information to it. Many websites offer impartial advice and information that has been compiled and checked by qualified medical professionals. Some, on the other hand, are run by commercial organisations with the purpose of promoting their own products. Others still are run by pressure groups, some of which will provide carefully assessed and accurate information whereas others may be suggesting medications or treatments that are not supported by the medical and scientific community.

Unless you know the address of the website you want to visit – for example, www.familydoctor.co.uk – you may find the following guidelines useful when searching the internet for information.

Search engines and other searchable sites

Google (www.google.co.uk) is the most popular search engine used in the UK, followed by Yahoo! (http://uk.yahoo.com) and MSN (www.msn.co.uk). Also popular are the search engine provided by Internet Service Providers such as TalkTalk and other sites such as the BBC site (www.bbc.co.uk).

In addition to the search engines that index the whole web, there are also medical sites with search facilities, which act almost like mini-search engines, but cover only medical topics or even a particular area of medicine. Again, it is wise to look at who is responsible for compiling the information offered to ensure that it is impartial and medically accurate. The NHS Direct site (www.nhsdirect.nhs.uk) is an example of a searchable medical site.

Links to many British medical charities can be found at the Association of Medical Research Charities website (www.amrc.org.uk) and at Charity Choice (www.charitychoice.co.uk).

Search phrases

Be specific when entering a search phrase. Searching for information on 'cancer' will return results for many different types of cancer as well as on cancer in general. You may even find sites offering astrological information. More useful results will be returned by using search phrases such as 'lung cancer' and 'treatments for lung cancer'. Both Google and Yahoo! offer an advanced search option that includes the ability to search for the exact phrase, enclosing the search phrase in quotes, that is, 'treatments for lung cancer' will have the same effect. Limiting a search to an exact phrase reduces the number of results returned but it is best to refine a search to an exact match only if you are not getting useful results with a normal search. Adding 'UK' to your search term will bring up mainly British sites, so a good phrase might be 'lung cancer' UK (don't include UK within the quotes).

Always remember the internet is international and unregulated. It holds a wealth of valuable information but individual sites may be biased, out of date or just plain wrong. Family Doctor Publications accepts no responsibility for the content of links published in this series.

Index

Your pages

We have included the following pages because they may help you manage your illness or condition and its treatment.

Before an appointment with a health professional, it can be useful to write down a short list of questions of things that you do not understand, so that you can make sure that you do not forget anything.

Some of the sections may not be relevant to your circumstances.

We are always pleased to receive constructive criticism or suggestions about how to improve the books. You can contact us at:

Email: familydoctor@btinternet.com
Letter: Family Doctor Publications
         PO Box 4664
         Poole
         BH15 1NN

Thank you

Health-care contact details

Name:

Job title:

Place of work:

Tel:

Name:

Job title:

Place of work:

Tel:

Name:

Job title:

Place of work:

Tel:

Name:

Job title:

Place of work:

Tel:

Significant past health events – illnesses/ operations/investigations/treatments

Event	Month	Year	Age (at time)

Appointments for health care

Name:

Place:

Date:

Time:

Tel:

Name:

Place:

Date:

Time:

Tel:

Name:

Place:

Date:

Time:

Tel:

Name:

Place:

Date:

Time:

Tel:

Appointments for health care

Name:

Place:

Date:

Time:

Tel:

Name:

Place:

Date:

Time:

Tel:

Name:

Place:

Date:

Time:

Tel:

Name:

Place:

Date:

Time:

Tel:

Current medication(s) prescribed by your doctor

Medicine name:
_____

Purpose:
_____

Frequency & dose:
_____

Start date:
_____

End date:
_____

Medicine name:
_____

Purpose:
_____

Frequency & dose:
_____

Start date:
_____

End date:
_____

Medicine name:
_____

Purpose:
_____

Frequency & dose:
_____

Start date:
_____

End date:
_____

Medicine name:
_____

Purpose:
_____

Frequency & dose:
_____

Start date:
_____

End date:
_____

Other medicines/supplements you are taking, not prescribed by your doctor

Medicine/treatment:

Purpose:

Frequency & dose:

Start date:

End date:

Medicine/treatment:

Purpose:

Frequency & dose:

Start date:

End date:

Medicine/treatment:

Purpose:

Frequency & dose:

Start date:

End date:

Medicine/treatment:

Purpose:

Frequency & dose:

Start date:

End date:

Questions to ask at appointments
(Note: do bear in mind that doctors work under great time pressure, so long lists may not be helpful for either of you)

Questions to ask at appointments
(Note: do bear in mind that doctors work under great time
pressure, so long lists may not be helpful for either of you)

Notes